Narrative Research in Nursing

Immy Holloway

Dawn Freshwater

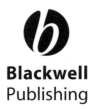

Blackwell
Publishing

© 2007 by Immy Holloway and Dawn Freshwater

Blackwell Publishing editorial offices:
Blackwell Publishing Ltd, 9600 Garsington Road, Oxford OX4 2DQ, UK
Tel: +44 (0)1865 776868
Blackwell Publishing Inc., 350 Main Street, Malden, MA 02148-5020, USA
Tel: +1 781 388 8250
Blackwell Publishing Asia Pty Ltd, 550 Swanston Street, Carlton, Victoria 3053, Australia
Tel: +61 (0)3 8359 1011

First published 2007 by Blackwell Publishing Ltd

ISBN: 978-1-4051-1408-0

Library of Congress Cataloging-in-Publication Data
Holloway, Immy. Narrative research in nursing / Immy Holloway, Dawn Freshwater.
p. ; cm.
Includes bibliographical references and index.
ISBN: 978-1-4051-1408-0 (pbk. : alk. paper)
1. Nursing—Research. 2. Discourse analysis, Narrative. I. Freshwater, Dawn. II. Title.
[DNLM: 1. Nursing Research—methods. 2. Narration. WY 20.5 H745n 2007]
RT81.5.H65 2007
610.73072—dc22
2006022222

A catalogue record for this title is available from the British Library

Set in 10/12.5 pt Palatino
by Graphicraft Limited, Hong Kong
Printed and bound in Singapore
by Markono Print Media Pte Ltd

The publisher's policy is to use permanent paper from mills that operate a
sustainable forestry policy, and which has been manufactured from pulp processed
using acid-free and elementary chlorine-free practices. Furthermore, the publisher
ensures that the text paper and cover board used have met acceptable environmental
accreditation standards.

For further information on Blackwell Publishing, visit our website:
www.blackwellnursing.com

Contents

Preface

Narrative research has increasingly been used in the social sciences, particularly in education, and is much advocated in nursing inquiry, be it in research with patients, colleagues and other health professionals or, indeed, in nurse education.

Narratives are accounts of experiences over time within an overall plot with a beginning, middle and end, though not always told sequentially. Rather like the experience of being a patient, a nurse or a researcher, the narrative plot is highly dependent upon the context. The notion of emplotment is something that has been explored in depth in literary criticism and is only now beginning to be examined in the light of narrative research (see for example Ricoeur, 1984) and nursing practice (Freshwater and Rolfe, 2004). Narrative data are collected through listening to the patients' stories about their experiences and interpretations of an illness, treatment or care. Data could also be obtained in nurse education from students or colleagues as well as in clinical settings from peers and other professionals. The analysis of these data can be used to improve patient care, interaction between professionals, and nursing education.

Researchers need listening skills during the in-depth, narrative interviews used in this approach. They elicit narratives from the participants in the study. Auto/biographical research belongs to this genre as does life story research. Although the approach stands on its own, it can also be used as part of other approaches (such as phenomenology and auto-ethnography). These issues and the different ways of doing narrative research are discussed in our book. All this is set in the cultural context of research. Narrativity is an emerging method, and one which places the voices of the 'researched' as central to the research process. This might explain the increasing enthusiasm in nursing for research approaches that embrace narrative methods. However, it is also important to acknowledge the level of disenchantment and disillusionment in nursing with the dominance of the evidence model that acts as the drive for evidence based practice and clinical effectiveness; narratives present a different kind of evidence.

We explore the analysis of data within the text specifically from the narrative viewpoint. Ethical issues are discussed and developed; the rigour and authenticity of this type of research have to be examined too. We explore the critique and problems inherent in narrative inquiry and give possible solutions to the problems proposed. Finally, we hope that the book will help others to write and publish narrative research and to consider the variety of media that can be utilised in presenting it.

We would encourage experienced researchers to select chapters appropriate to their needs, while suggesting that the novice researcher might benefit from reading the whole book.

The aim and readership of the book

The text is mainly addressed to nurses, be they academics or students who are undertaking either undergraduate or postgraduate studies that require knowledge of research. It is not intended for complete novices in research but for those who already know a little about qualitative approaches. It could also be useful for practitioners wishing to carry out narrative inquiry in clinical practice.

This is a book about a specific way of research for nursing. Other health professionals too might find it useful. It is fair to reflect that the concepts which are incorporated within the narrative approach are transferable both across geographical areas and across professional boundaries.

Acknowledgements

We would like to thank our editor, Beth Knight, for her help and encouragement and Philip Esterhuizen for his insights into narrative ethics.

About the Authors

Immy Holloway is a Professor and Co-director of the Centre for Qualitative Research (with Les Todres) in the Institute of Health and Community Studies at Bournemouth University. As a medical sociologist she is particularly interested in qualitative approaches in the field of health research. She has published extensively in this area and is the author of several books which have been translated into foreign languages.

Dawn Freshwater is a Professor of nursing research at Murdoch University and is Director of the Centre for Applied Research in Mental Health at Bournemouth University. Her interests are in reflexive, narrative and deconstructive approaches to research and development. She has authored/co-authored and edited 14 books, some of which have been translated into other languages. She is a Fellow of the Royal College of Nursing, Editor of the *Journal of Psychiatric and Mental Health Nursing* and current President of the International Association for Human Caring.

Perspectives on
Narrative Research

1 The Nature and Features of Narrative Research

Narrative research is now a frequently used way of carrying out qualitative research and has gained in popularity recently. It is located at the end of a continuum of forms of inquiry which range from various types of qualitative research in which the researcher is fully in control, through structured or semi-structured modes of observation and interviews, to the unstructured methods of narrative inquiry where participants have much control over the process of the research. However, there is no consensus about the nature of narrative research (Ollerenshaw and Creswell, 2002) although it exists in various forms which will be discussed later. The type of narrative research that we discuss in this book is not specific (as in phenomenology) but covers narrative inquiry and analysis in general. The ever increasing use of narrative in research – and practice – is often called 'the narrative turn' in human sciences.

Carrying out narrative research is doing both art and science: making art is a creative act concerned with generating an effect – be it beauty or surprise. The artistic goal in narrative research adds creative, aesthetic and craft elements, but it also enhances practice. Its main strength lies in its communicative power and its immediacy. Researchers participating in it also engage their emotions, and they are not neutral or distant but empathic and close to the narrators. This research is also science – albeit social or human science. Mason (2002) counters the arguments of quantitative researchers who, when applying 'scientific criteriology', do not see qualitative research as scientific. She claims that the criteria by which science is judged are in themselves problematic. This type of research cannot be forced into a single set of prescriptions, principles and rules, but it is methodical and systematic. Science, after all, is knowledge gained through systematic procedures and processes in empirical study, but in qualitative research – and narrative research is one approach within the qualitative continuum – it is not seen as generating, testing and refuting or confirming hypotheses. Reason (2003: 206) sees the science of persons as an attempt to move 'beyond grand narratives toward localized, practical knowings that are based in experience . . .'. All scientific research, whether in the natural or social sciences, demands a critical stance on one's own discoveries and a rigorous approach. It does need evidence; in narrative research it is produced and demonstrated in a different way from that in natural science inquiry. Harré (2004) in fact states that qualitative research is scientific because it has reflexivity, meaning and specificity. *Reflexivity* demands that the writer be reflective about the reflections of the participants. Harré calls this second-level reflection and maintains that this contributes to the scientific character of the research. Another element of science is the generation of the *meaning* of experience and the manner in which it is represented to others. Science is also inherent in the *specificity* of the work of researchers.

Nurses carrying out research increasingly use narratives of patients and colleagues to explore phenomena that interest them. Through narratives they wish to study the experience of people in context. Before describing narrative research in nursing, however, we shall attempt a definition and discussion of the concept 'narrative'.

Defining the concept and character of narrative

Narratives are 'a basic and universal mode of human expression' (Smith, 2000: 327). According to Labov and Waletzky (1967: 12) they are 'the oral versions of personal experience', although written versions also exist in autobiographies and life histories, for instance. These writers demanded specific and necessary elements in narratives: such as an *abstract* as a summary of the narrative, *orientation* such as that of time, location and participants, *complicating action* – the events that took place, the *evaluation* of the latter, the final *resolution* and *coda*, but this might be seen as a prescriptive approach to story analysis.

The description and analysis approach of Labov and Waletzky has sometimes been seen as too rigid and heavily structured as well as complex (Elliott, 2005). In their simplest form narratives are continuous stories with connected elements that include a plot, a stated problem and a cast of characters. The story is generally a verbal or written representation of events or experiences, expressed in a way that can be understood by others, while a plot, according to Sarbin (1986: 3), is 'a recognizable pattern of events'. Stories include the element of temporality, that is, they are placed within a time span and often link the present to the past and the future. Indeed, time and sequence are some of narrative's most important features. The core narrative tells the listener what it's all about and is the narrator's interpretation of the story's point. Narratives are always about something, for instance illness, or disability, or treatment, or everyday life. Freeman (2003: 335) calls this referential element in narrative 'aboutness'.

Another, more complex definition of narrative is that by Polkinghorne (1988: 13): 'Narrative is the fundamental scheme for linking individual human actions and events into interrelated aspects of an understandable composite.' The concept 'narrative' contains a multiplicity of meanings; indeed it is an overall term, and single or precise definitions are difficult. Frank (1995) makes a distinction between the concepts of story and narrative. He cites the term 'story' when discussing the tales people tell, and 'narrative' when referring to general structures encompassing a number of particular stories. However, the line is blurred, and often these concepts are used interchangeably though the terms differ in their semantic roots. The word 'narrative' derives from the Latin *gnarus* meaning knowing, while 'story' comes from the Greek and Latin *historia* which also means knowing (by inquiry) as well as an account of events. Etymological dictionaries also inform us that *histos* means web or tissue; this illuminates the words 'history' and 'story' in an interesting way. Researchers now often prefer to use the terms 'narrative' and 'story' as synonymous. An imaginative explanation that has resonance with health professionals is that by Connelly and Clandinin (1990), two educational researchers, quoted in Cortazzi (1993: 17): 'Narrative refers to the making of meaning through personal experience by way of a process of reflection in which storytelling is a key element and in which metaphors and folk knowledge take their place.'

There is more than one approach to the study of narrative. Phenomenologists, discourse analysts, grounded theorists and other qualitative researchers use narrative interviewing to obtain data generated by narratives and build their research on the participants' stories. Indeed these researchers retell – re-story – or rewrite the narratives of the participants in research in various ways. This means that they often – though not always – go through a process of interpretation. Narratives are sources of data in psychology, sociology and anthropology, and those disciplines that are informed by social science such as nursing, medicine and education (Clandinin and Connelly, 2000; Hurwitz et al., 2004), but the significance of narrative was of course initially recognised in literature and fits in the literary tradition as well as social science. The study of narrative has broadened out from its use in literature, and is now used for analysis of experience and events in other areas such as the social sciences and health care. Indeed, Lieblich et al. (1998: 2) state that narrative research 'refers to any study that uses or analyses narrative material'.

In this book, we shall use the singular and plural of narrative as Polkinghorne (1988: 8) intended it: 'narrative' is the form or process of telling stories, while 'narratives' refers to the unique stories of individuals, which are distinct in content and plot. Narratives, in the sense discussed in this book, are personal accounts of people's motives, experiences and actions, and the way they interpret and assign meanings to them. They do not consist merely of single statements or phrases but are lengthy accounts and reflections of the narrator, the person who tells the story and who translates experience and reflection on actions and behaviour into language in order to communicate it to others. All human beings tell others of their experience in the form of stories and, through using language, shape and transform it. Narrative is a holistic presentation of that experience. Indeed, Clandinin and Connelly (2000) see experience as the starting point and core of narrative research. Persons, time, actions and events are embedded in the stories that individuals share with each other.

When academics spoke of narrative in the past, they referred to the grand narrative in and of literature, often neglecting the everyday story of ordinary folk. Now they focus more on local knowledge and the vividness and plausibility of this type of story, and value all people's storytelling.

Narrative in a historical context

The idea of narrative goes back to ancient times, to the 'Poetics' of Aristotle according to Bruner (2002). Bruner also suggests that Propp, a folklorist in Russia, started the study of narrative in the 20th century. In its modern form the term has been used particularly from the mid 20th century in linguistics, literary criticism and phenomenology – especially phenomenological psychology – as well as in anthropology and sociology. It is also often used in psychotherapy. Language is the main tool of communication through which people are able to illuminate their experience, and express their identity and their perceptions of culture. Häninnen (2004), a psychologist, differentiates between different modes of narrativity, namely the *told narrative*, the *inner narrative* and the *lived narrative*. The first of these refers to what researchers often use for analysis. As noted previously, it is spoken or written and usually autobiographical; it is also closely linked to culture. This type of story reflects and makes explicit the ongoing inner narrative. However, the told and inner narratives also interact in other ways: the told narrative has an effect on, and shapes, the inner narrative. The former, however, is intended to have an effect on the listener and hence is more dramatic and includes – perhaps – more justification of behaviour. Researchers, of course, have to rely for their inquiry on the told narrative, which may or may not be 'the whole story'.

The inner narrative, Häninnen suggests, is that which centres on the story that human beings tell themselves, and which organises their experiences. It gives direction to both actions and words because it contains elements of the individual's morality, values and goals; although it depends on language, it is not wholly verbal. There is a strong link between a person's situation in culture and time and the inner narrative, as individuals formulate the narrative according to their standpoint and choose from a variety of alternative stories that fit into their cultural framework.

The lived narrative focuses on the narrative character of human life as people live their lives in narrative form: that is, they act out a succession of narrative episodes. In research, however, these three forms of narrative overlap and interact. The stories of events that people tell to outsiders are possibly less deep and rich than inner narrative which is part of their identity and the interpretation of what happens to them as well as giving meaning to action. Both, however, are reflections on and representations of the 'lived experience'. The told narrative makes explicit in words some of the elements of the other forms of narrative. The lived narrative acts out the inner narrative, according to Häninnen; it guides individuals' behaviour and the interaction with others. Researchers must be aware of how these modes of narrative interact with each other.

'The narrative turn' in the social sciences is not part of the literary tradition but is acquiring its own tradition and conventions, and it is seen as an important change in the last few decades. Writers do not often acknowledge or recognise the origin of narrative in literary theory except for the narratologists of the recent past, as Hyvärinen (2004) claims. She speaks of a 'transition from a mode of representation to a metaphor of life' (p. 3). However, she also states that small stories about a section of people's lives – such as an illness for instance – seem to replace whole life stories or autobiographical tales.

The sociologists Labov and Waletzky wrote a now classic article on 'narrative analysis' in 1966 and published it in 1967; they perceived narrative as a way of creating meaning from the unexpected. These authors take a structural approach to narratives which is sometimes criticised as inappropriate for the genre (Parker, 2004).

Life stories, and educational, illness and professional narratives, have been popular since the 1980s [for instance in the work of Sarbin (1986), Mishler (1991), Josselson and Lieblich (1993) and Riessman (1993)]. In nursing and other forms of health care, they have been widely used in the late 20th century and the early years of the 21st. Narrative approaches also include autobiography, autoethnography, biography and oral history according to Alvermann (2000). The terms are self-explanatory, but we shall come back to them in the discussion of data sources.

Telling tales

Narration is part of human nature, and people have a natural desire to share stories of experience and communicate what they feel and think.

Although there is a debate about whether narrative structures are inherent or acquired through culture (Polkinghorne, 1988), this is not of interest for those who carry out health research. They merely ask: what use are stories in the generation of knowledge about phenomena in the area of health care?

Human beings narrate past events and experience all through their lives from childhood onwards to 'inform, instruct, entertain, empower, exonerate or cathart, among other things' (Smith, 2000: 327). Narratives are more holistic accounts than the fractured answers that participants might give to interview questions. Polkinghorne (1995) does not like the term 'story' as he feels that it sounds as though the narrative might not be true and could be linked to something made up by the narrator, and thus have connotations of 'falsely constructed experience' (see Chapter 4). Bruner (1986), however, states that although stories do not necessarily depend on empirical verification, they are still versions of reality: the social reality as seen by the narrator. When people tell their own story, they reflect on the meaning and significance of their experience, and through this construct and reconstruct their identities (see Chapter 4).

Bruner (1986) suggests that narrative reasoning is one of the two main methods of human cognition: the other is scientific reasoning. He does not criticise the way we acquire knowledge through science; indeed he places expository and paradigmatic (as he calls it) cognition on an equal basis with narrative knowledge. The two are, in his view, merely different forms of knowing, though they are equally valid. In research, particularly in the past, stories have often been seen as subordinate to scientific reports, and formal language was valued more highly than more personal and narrative language. This has changed in the last decade. The knowledge acquired through narratives encapsulates human motivation, that is, why people behave as they do. Whereas researchers who use paradigmatic cognition search for generalisations and often test or verify hypotheses, those who work in the narrative inquiry mode gain knowledge from individual and unique cases from which they cannot generalise, though similarities and patterns might be recognised. Bruner (1991) argues that the memory of events and the organisation of experience are mediated through narratives, and that individuals tell stories in their own way depending on culture and significant others. These stories are people's versions of reality and not scientific constructions, but they also give 'evidence' of what individuals feel and think; hence narrative research too is evidence based.

Through storytelling, disparate parts of experience become integrated into a whole and events and happenings are organised and connected. People wish to make sense of this experience by telling a coherent, contextualised story embedded in their feelings. They also include judgements, appraisals, assessments and reasons.

Human lives are lived through narrative, and the history of human-kind is littered with stories. This type of, mainly verbal, representation is, as Kreiswirth (2000) acknowledges, embedded in human consciousness and part of everyday life and discourse. It is, of course, debatable whether researchers can claim narrative as part of 'human sciences' (*Geisteswissenschaften* or *sciences humaines*) which generates new knowledge. Its exact character and working process have yet to be presented clearly.

The social and cultural context of stories

The culture of the storytellers affects the stories they tell, and therefore a person does not operate in a 'cultural vacuum' in Bruner's (1991: 20) words. Narrative as a social process connects to issues of culture and power. Cultural concepts and beliefs provide a framework for individuals in which they can become narrators of their story, and social positioning influences their storytelling. Narratives generate 'local knowledge' because of their link to social context and unique experience in time rather than universal statements that can be applied everywhere and forever.

In our society, health professionals are seen as members of an élite culture. Their clients do often believe in and follow the dominant discourse of health professionals, employers, or even researchers in health care and research settings. In storytelling, however, participants in narrative inquiry have the power to define their own bodies, identities and experience, rather than having their reality shaped by others. People are active agents in their own experience, not passive recipients; they are able to assert themselves, 'recover agency', and achieve self-esteem.

The cultural framework is nevertheless not the only factor that influences storytellers in spite of its strength and pervasiveness. There is also the uniquely personal and individual effect of the self of a storyteller as well as the influence of the specific situation in which persons find themselves that is affected by culture but by no means wholly determined by it. The individual is an active human being who can determine – within social and cultural boundaries – his or her own story.

Narrative, plot and emplotment

Story, narrative and plot are closely related and often, in the literature at least, confused and conflated (Cobley, 2004; see also Freshwater and

Rolfe, 2004). These three fundamentally separate aspects of a narration clearly blend in a 'pleasing way', but, as Cobley (2004) illustrates, have subtle distinctions.

In an attempt to clarify the difference between story, plot and narrative, Cobley (2004: 5) uses a contemporary media lens as opposed to technical definitions. Simply explained, story, he argues, consists of 'all the events which are to be depicted'. Perhaps one might think of this as the 'what' of the narrative, whilst plot is 'the chain of causation which dictates that these events are somehow linked and that they are therefore to be depicted in relation to each other'. The plot, then, is the circumstance which brings the character to life through a specific series of events; a chain of causality that creates meaning and structure through emplotment. In contrast, narrative 'is the showing or the telling of these events and the mode selected for that to take place' (Cobley, 2004: 6). We could frame this view of narrative as the 'how' of the narration; how the story is told; how the story is presented; and how the characters are represented.

Not all writers agree with Cobley (2004) and others on their distinction between story, plot and narrative (see, for example, Chatman, 1978; Wiltshire, 1995). Narrative (research/researchers) does not necessarily reveal the plot in a temporal sequence, and it is selective in its choice of events, omitting some and including others. Here we include the researcher and research, for whilst every narrative requires a sequence, the way in which that sequence becomes meaningful is through human interaction, be that through the writer, reader, researcher or listener. Cobley (2004: 8) captures this succinctly, stating: 'A sequence of any kind might exist in the world, but if that sequence is to consist of meaningful relations it requires human input.' Such sequencing is heavily reliant on concepts of time and space, which, according to French philosopher Paul Ricoeur (1984), are intimately related to narrative; in fact he argues that narrative is the human relation to time. We will return to the relevance of temporality and spatiality at various points throughout the text. The work of Ricoeur is of significance when discussing the relationship between narrative, plot and emplotment, to which we now turn.

According to Ricoeur (1984), plot or emplotment is the cornerstone of narrative structure. Moreover, it is the intelligible whole governing the succession of events in a story. White (1973) argues that plot is not found, rather it is made. In his work on *metahistory* he notes that most modern stories are emplotted with classical tropes – figures of speech, the four main ones (or master tropes) being metaphor, metonymy, synecdoche and irony. Tropes, which permeate all linguistic expression, are also linked to dramaturgical conventions, such as those traditionally found within a European culture: romance, comedy, satire and tragedy. This repertoire of classical plots is very familiar, and although new themes and concepts might be overlaid, it is often the case that the classical plot remains transparent. That is to say that these classical (and culturally embedded) plots are both resistant and resilient, even in the face of enormous societal and historical revolution.

Emplotment is central to the building and development of a story; it is the structure through which sense is made of events and the way in which things are connected (Czarniawska, 2004; Freshwater and Rolfe, 2004). Ryan (1993) points out that whilst what is happening in the story (the chronicle) and how the story is painted to the listener or reader (the mimesis) are important dimensions of the way a story is constructed, it is in fact the emplotment that is the real challenge and, as we interpret, the craft: that is, the linking of the events into a meaningful sequence and structure. It is natural, of course, for the audience, whoever they may be, to want to create their own emplotment in response to the story. Plot, then, is a device of narrative. Despite the emphasis on time and space in narrative by Ricoeur and others, Czarniawska (2004: 125) reminds us that temporal and spatial connections are not sufficient to act as a plot. She notes that: 'To become a plotted story, the elements, or episodes, need also to be related by *transformation*'. This could be related to linking of narrative, plot, authority and reflexivity in the chapter 'The Event of a Narrative' by Freshwater and Rolfe (2004), which does not explicitly refer to transformation; rather the authors emphasise the notion of power and freedom afforded through narrative to expose the limitations and constraints of old meanings and old plots.

Of course Ricoeur's own views of narrative have changed over time, an example itself of the interdependence of time and narrative. More recently, he has focused on the activity that produces the plot, rather than the plot itself. Parallels could be drawn with reflexivity here, in that reflexive researchers are not overly concerned with the content of the research, rather they are interested in the making of that content (Freshwater, 2006). This distinction between the process and the content of a narrative will be further explored in other chapters, where we examine the practice of narrative analysis through examining content, structure and form and how the text performs.

Greenhalgh and Hurwitz (1998: 4) suggest a difference between a simple story and a plot, taking their suggestion from E.M. Forster's (1927) explanation that a simple story continues in a chronology '. . . and then . . . and then . . .', while the plot suggests 'why' (causation will be discussed later). Plot is the sequential element and the essential structure of narrative (Cortazzi, 1993) as we have suggested. Plotlines, however, are not always linear; they may be circular or iterative and can be revised or 'edited' in their retelling. Going back and forth is quite common among narrators but the listener is still left with the essential features of the story. Researchers attempt to find the 'narrative thread' to grasp the whole story and give it coherence.

The narrative is a journey or pathway through time which is told by its author, who tells the listener what happens on the way. The narrator takes a reflective stance on events and processes on the journey. However, narrators do not merely communicate a simple story to the listener; they also clarify and reflect on the past and justify their past behaviour and link the past to their present thinking and actions. Brody (2003) adds to these features of narrative another element: the story has to be special, that is, 'worthy' of narration. It doesn't rely merely on everyday sequences of events: 'I took the car; I drove to work; I talked to my friends.' Instead it relies on dramatic and critical events and behaviour, when critical events or situations are discussed such as an unusual condition, an illness or an epiphany where some thing or person is illuminated by a sudden insight: 'I was digging in the garden, and all of a sudden I felt a snap in my back. The pain was excruciating . . .'.

As we have already mentioned, the term emplotment describes the way a story is organised. Cortazzi (1993) describes three major elements in a plot, some of which are mentioned by Ricoeur (1984) also:

(1) Temporality
(2) Causation
(3) Human interest

Temporality

Temporality implies that the story evolves more or less sequentially (although this could be disputed). It means that there are three linked sequences: when the story is set up and opens up towards the future – the beginning; when the story unfolds – the middle; when the story is resolved – the end. For instance:

> I was digging in the garden for an hour, and then I went into the house; after a while I noticed that my back hurt terribly.

The listener can hear that the story has coherence because the narrator links past, present and future. Indeed, even in a dramatic and chaotic story, the listener can detect plot and coherence, though Freeman (2003) suggests that narratives are more chaotic than is sometimes assumed as lives themselves are not necessarily coherent and structured.

Causation

A story often contains causal relationships, which listeners and readers generally perceive even though they are often assumed. For instance:

I was digging in the garden for an hour, and then I went into the house; after a while I noticed that my back hurt terribly.

The audience understands this as: 'My digging caused the back pain I experienced.'

As human beings we are constructed in such a way that we continually search for the causes of things. Story, with its inherent linearity, provides a powerful experience of causation, gratifying this basic need. Porter Abbott (2002: 37) suggests that 'narrative itself, simply by the way it distributes events in an orderly, consecutive fashion, very often gives the impression of a sequence of cause and effect'. Forster (2005), in his definitive text *Aspects of the Novel*, gives some practical examples of the way in which readers do not always need causation to be obvious in a text in order to think causally. In other words human beings have a tendency towards a narrative logic, in which things that follow other things are caused by those things. Barthes (1982), however, challenges the notion of narrative logic (which he describes as a fallacy), stating that the confusion between consecution and consequence is the mainspring of narrative and leads to bad social science. Porter Abbott (2002), however, questions whether narratives must show a cause: that is, whether cause is a defining feature of a narrative, or if narrative is the representation of events not necessarily bound by causal links. A further question, then, and one that we return to in Chapter 8, concerns the relationship between causality and narrative analysis/interpretation. To what extent does the researcher ascribe causation to the narrative through their individual interpretation and in the analytic process (Freshwater and Avis, 2004)?

Human interest

Human interest is another element in the story. If no one has an interest in the story, then there is no listener and no narrative. Often a story of experience includes crises and turning points as well as justification for the storyteller's actions and behaviour that are a response to the interpretation of experience. Jovchelovitch and Bauer (2000) also discuss the dimensions of stories: the chronological, which involves time and sequence, and the non-chronological, in which researchers construct a plot from separate events forming a coherent whole.

Illness narratives

Finally there needs to be a discussion of stories of sickness, or as Kleinman (1988) calls them: 'Illness Narratives' (followed up in

Chapter 3). These are stories people tell about their illness or perceived condition. Kleinman wrote a foundational text on this type of story, much used by health professionals but also criticised. He claims that health professionals can learn about suffering and vulnerability by studying the illness experiences of their clients. These stories demonstrate how patients make sense of their situation and condition. However, they also show how patients perceive their treatment, and how they adapt to problems and cope with their situation. The reaction of health professionals and significant others to their condition and story becomes part of their perception. Nurses usually have closer and more intimate contact with patients and therefore are often the first audience to listen to these illness narratives. Kleinman (p. 9) suggests that 'the interpretation of meaning can also contribute to the provision of more effective care.' Greenhalgh and Hurwitz (1998) too add, in their text on narrative-based medicine, that narratives can provide clues and generate understanding between health professionals and clients. They claim that listening can topple long-held assumption and 'challenge received wisdom' and thus go beyond 'facts' in the clinical encounter while providing the meaning which clients attach to their conditions. Illness narratives also point to power relationships in the sense that social structure and hierarchy are reflected in them; people feel in control or powerless, depending on their perception of their location in the social setting.

Narratives are an expression of people's identity which might become threatened during illness and adversity. Indeed, Bury (2001: 264) claims that in times of 'biographical disruption', after problematic and adverse experiences, human beings re-mould their narratives 'to maintain a sense of identity' (revisited in Chapter 4).

Summary

We began this chapter by referring to the 'narrative turn' in the human sciences. In defining the basic concepts of narrative, story, plot and emplotment, we have attempted to highlight some of the wide-ranging and far-reaching meanings and interpretations of narrative within the literature. In this sense, the definitions of these concepts mirror the event of narrative itself; that is to say that narrative is open to multiple interpretations. Narrative is part of human nature; narrative research is closely associated with understanding people's lives rather than abstract principles. Illness narratives can also be the focus of health professionals' concern.

2 Narrative Research: Understanding People's Lives

Through first-person stories, health professionals are able to gain greater understanding of patients. This contributes to more effective care and treatment. Narrative research, however, is used in a different way from practice narratives, although the ultimate aims of both types of narrative are similar.

Narrative inquiry in health care means that participant narratives are used for research purposes. It is concerned with people's lives and experiences, as the term implies, and examines the ways in which individuals and cultural members construct their world. It is person-centred and generally linked to qualitative methodology, to the auto-biographical, to subjectivity and reflexivity, to culture and also to power. Josselson and Lieblich (2001) maintain that, through access to living in a common culture, narrative researchers are able to comprehend the complex process of human experience in the societal, cultural and historical context. It is, however, wise to bear in mind that researchers do not always share the cultural (or subcultural) framework of the participants and may misinterpret on the basis of their own assumptions.

Storytelling involves an audience, and storytellers narrate their tale to the researcher. Researchers in their turn retell the story to the reader of the research account. This means that the story is told several times over, evolving each time. Ollerenshaw and Creswell (2002: 332) claim that both the original narrator and the researcher are present in the text: 'Collaboration in narrative research means that the inquirer actively involves the participants in the inquiry as it unfolds.' The participants also actively involve the researcher in the story as it evolves. Through this the listeners meet the narrator and absorb what the storyteller has to say and respond to it while integrating it into their own understanding as well as filtering and interpreting it. As researchers we can, of course, examine what participants tell us and interpret it whilst being faithful to the original stories. As Riessman says (1993: 1): 'Storytelling, to put the argument simply, is what we do with our research materials, and what informants do with us.' Stories are the raw data of research and make the experiences of the participants its focus, but the stories become transformed in the process of both telling and listening. They are not just raw data but also interpretations of the researchers, and hence products of their thinking, interpretations and abstractions. Polkinghorne (1988) enumerates three main levels of narrative: experience, telling and interpreting. One could add to this the important action of listening, for without hearing the story it cannot be retold.

For instance, when men admit to losing their jobs through pain or illness, they do not always explicitly state that they have lost their masculine roles in a society that values breadwinners. The researcher infers and states this change in role relationships while interpreting the tale of loss.

Typologies, models and features of narrative

Writers have attempted to construct a typology of narrative (for instance, Richardson, 1990; Frank, 1995; Mishler, 1995). Richardson discusses five major types of narrative:

(1) The everyday story
(2) The autobiographical story
(3) The biographical story
(4) The cultural story
(5) The collective story

The everyday story involves time and continuance. People tell each other about the experience of their day or week, how they spent their time, what happened to them during this time. This connects them with others who have similar experiences, 'linking the personal to the public' (p. 125).

The example below is an illustration of an everyday story about the day of a person in chronic pain. This part of a story demonstrates how a person fits in a routine day, in spite of feeling unwell.

'When I get up I always experience a great deal of pain and I take it slowly. After breakfast when I feel more mobile, my husband takes me to the shops . . . and then I might do some gardening in the afternoon.' (A woman with chronic back pain)

The autobiographical story connects the present with the past and the future. The narrative is one of individual history and biography and helps people to come to terms with what happened to them during the course of time. An example is shown below:

'I have this very rare form of leukaemia. The consultant initially said that there are so many forms of it, that it is not certain which form of chemotherapy would help it. I have always been such a healthy person, and I've had such a healthy lifestyle: how is it possible to get something like this? I feel so unwell and depressed, but I do hope that I feel better in the future. I want to lead a full life as I'm still young, and I do hope that my condition lets me live long enough to achieve my personal ambitions to travel. I've always wanted to travel, and now it seems it is too late.'

Through autobiographical stories individuals attempt to establish themselves as distinguishable and separate from others and to make sense of their own lives, and they justify their actions. They also link the past to the present and future. The biographical story sees the world from other people's point of view. It is most often used in literary work such as novels or in biographies. The biographical story connects individuals with each other through intersubjectivity, because they share feelings and are empathetic with others. Nurses sometimes tell stories of an inspiring patient whom they remember. While reading the nurses' accounts or listening to them, other health professionals can share and compare experiences.

Through cultural stories people make visible meanings in a particular social context (Holloway and Wheeler, 2002). They link the story to the understandings that exist in a culture about a specific condition or disability. 'My friend has AIDS. I wouldn't tell anybody about it because it is still a shameful condition in this country and people would be afraid to go to the pub with him.' Or 'The doctor doesn't really know whether to believe that I'm in pain. Now, if I had a broken leg . . .'.

The following is an excerpt from a cultural story:

'My wife, she's took my role on,
and I've taken on hers,
and that can be really really hard . . .'

(Holloway et al., 2000)

The preceding story, told by a middle-aged labourer, is deeply bedded in a culture where the roles of males and females are still prescribed to a large extent. The tale told by a young professional person in Western culture might sound quite different. Richardson suggests that people have a general understanding of the meanings in a culture, and that the cultural story is 'embedded in larger cultural and social frameworks' (p. 127). However, one might suggest that most of our stories, particularly tales of suffering and illness, are influenced and sometimes even determined by the cultural and social environment.

The collective story also has elements of culture, autobiography and biography. It is, according to Richardson, the story of powerless and marginalised persons. They claim for themselves a social category to which they belong, such as 'the disabled', 'the suffering', 'the survivors of abuse'. People do tell the individual story, but they often link this to the narrative of others to demonstrate that they belong to a particular group.

Richardson suggests that collective stories have 'transformative possibilities'. Although people give meaning to their lives by telling stories within a cultural framework, they are able to deviate from the standard story by forming new narratives. Thus non-hearing or partially hearing people, for instance, do not always pressure the system to help them regain their hearing but maintain that 'being deaf' does not mean 'being disabled', and stress that society should come to terms with deaf people rather than changing them. Thus the condition 'being deaf' is transformed, and a new plot is created which affects the future of these individuals. The craft of emplotment is of significance to the researcher who, when working with narrative data, is focused not only on interpreting the plot in the data but also on emplotting that plot within a plot of their own through the research narrative. In other words, the research introduces a structure that enables the story, as it is reported, to make sense.

A number of common features are shared by narratives, and some of these are listed by Greenhalgh and Hurwitz (1998):

- Narrative has a finite time sequence
- Narrative implies a narrator and an audience
- Narrative is linked to the individual
- Narrative is based on the subjective experience of the storyteller
- Narrative is a story capable of holding the audience's interest

Narrative has a finite time sequence with a beginning, a middle and an end, as we said before. The middle contains a number of events and happenings which are unfolding in the telling of the story.

Narrative implies a narrator, the storyteller, and an audience that listens to the story. In narrative research this is initially at least the researcher. The narrative is linked to individuals, their experiences and feelings, and the way they understand their situation. Individuals are authors of their own stories. This means that the story is decided upon by the storytellers and does not necessarily describe events directly or in factual detail but depends on their subjective perspective of their experience. Nevertheless the stories are also linked to the cultural knowledge of the narrator and socially constructed. Individuals cannot separate themselves from their social context, their location in time, space and history. This means that the stories about a particular phenomenon, event or condition are similar and generate patterns, but each one is also unique at the same time. The authors of these stories might claim their uniqueness, but they are nevertheless embedded in the social and cultural context of the time in which they live. Josselson and Lieblich (2001: 281) state: 'The narrative researcher pays particular attention to aspects of the person's experience that relate to his or her socially constructed position in life, a position that might feel self-authored to the person but may actually be a product of the person's place in his or her culturally constituted world.' So although the story is an individual and unique construction, it is influenced – often without the knowledge of the storyteller – by location, time and culture; that is, stories of experience are not merely individualist projects but fit into a larger picture and demonstrate knowledge of the individual's location and time.

The narrative is a story in which the audience – or readership – can immerse itself and through which it can identify with the storyteller. Feelings experienced and knowledge acquired are transferred from the storyteller to the listener. This is only possible through intersubjective knowledge, knowledge which individuals share by inhabiting the same world; they understand by linking the knowledge acquired from the narrator to their own social reality, and thus researchers can become co-authors of the participants' stories when they present them in research reports. The process of telling stories leads to the product of the researcher narrative.

Bruner (1991) discusses the characteristics which he ascribes to narrative, and some of these will be discussed here. The first of these features is *diachronicity*. This means that the narrative account is of happenings occurring over time and has sequential elements. It is a pattern of events told in 'human time' and has duration. Bruner calls this time-boundedness 'sequenced durativity' (p. 6). *Particularity* is another characteristic of narrative. Although all stories fall into general types, narratives are also specific and this specificity is built into the general. For instance, there may be a general story of illness and loss, but it also has particularity as this illness can have specific elements and the loss may refer to the body or mental faculties. Events in people's lives are related to their lives in terms of belief systems, values and desires, and they express them in these terms. Everything in a narrative is there for the purpose for which it is intended. For instance, when discussing the actions of a nurse, a patient builds these into his or her beliefs or wishes. Meanings are expressed by people and extracted by listeners and readers. The researcher invites the reader into the story by making it as interesting as possible so that the reader is provided with access to people's lives. The participants' interpretations and those of the listeners are not, however, necessarily the same. Researchers cannot truly verify the whole of a story through conventional measures, nor the parts that constitute it; they must try instead to give a convincing report of the meaning of the whole illuminated by its constituent elements. *Hermeneutic composability* is a way of processing knowledge in an interpretive way. The narrator and the listener depend on their own background knowledge in their interpretation of the story. Bruner also stresses some of the features that others ascribe to narratives and their interpretations such as *context sensitivity* and *negotiability*. These show again that the background and culture of both storyteller and listener are important. There are often conflicting versions of one event across participants and between participants and the researcher. Thus the final version has to be negotiated between the participants and the researcher.

Another important feature is *narrative accrual*. Bruner suggests that people build up individual stories ('cobble stories together') and sets of similar stories into a whole. Eventually this accumulation becomes 'a culture' or 'a history' or 'a tradition' (p. 18). For instance, Kathryn Montgomery Hunter has composed a book of 'doctors' stories' (2001) which can be read as the description of a medical culture.

Social constructionism

Human beings are active in the construction of reality. They do not passively receive their view of the world from others – although other people, and in particular significant others – influence them. They are, instead, active agents in building their perspectives and perceptions of social reality within the context of their culture, locality and history. Culture, inclusive of language, roles and rules, becomes the filter through which individuals perceive their experiences and attach meaning to them. Meaning is shaped through social interaction and language. Many others are linked to the storytellers, namely significant others, all the members of the social group with whom they are connected, and the professionals with whom they interact. For instance, in telling their stories of illness, individuals are linked to family and friends, and those who treat and care for them. They make judgements about their illness and treatment, and share these with others. (We shall return to this topic in Chapter 4.)

The difference between narrative inquiry and other qualitative approaches

Narrative inquiry is an important genre within qualitative approaches, characterised mainly by its coherence and sequential form. These traits distinguish it from many other types of research. While much qualitative data collection results in 'fractured texts' (Riessman, 1993), narrative produces coherent stories.

The relationship and collaboration between researcher and researched is also different from other types of inquiry. Although there is an equality of relationship between the two protagonists in all qualitative inquiry – or at least that is one of its aims – in narrative research the participants have more power as they control the story to a large extent, and it is not guided by the researcher as it would be in a semi-structured interview. Participants link the narrative to the researcher's and reader's understanding and interpretation of the participants' reality. Researchers then connect the narratives to larger issues and the context of the social world.

For the purpose of this text we define 'narrative inquiry' as a distinct qualitative approach rather than seeing it as embedded within other qualitative approaches, although it may well be.

The functions of narratives

Why then do human beings tell stories, and why do researchers use narrative inquiry? Riessman (1993), Smith (2000) and Kellas and Manusov (2003) suggest a variety of reasons, and we shall list some of them here as well as adding our own. Reflections on experience may:

(1) Give meaning to and make sense of experience and emotions
(2) Help the narrator to interpret events
(3) Express, enhance or confirm the narrator's identity
(4) Segment and organise experience, actions and events
(5) Also provide a coherent whole of experience and thoughts
(6) Generate change in thinking through making explicit, and bring about adjustment to unalterable conditions
(7) Confirm group membership or group consciousness
(8) Attribute responsibility, blame or praise to specific individuals
(9) Allow individuals to take control of their own story

These functions of narrative will be illustrated when we discuss stories of illness and disability in a later chapter. Suffice to say that individuals are motivated to tell stories for a variety of reasons. Some of the elements above reveal the 'transformative' character of narrative. Telling stories enhances the freedom and control of individuals and understanding of their lives. In health and social care, stories are not told for the entertainment of others – although this may, rarely, be a by-product of research.

Järvinen (2004) maintains that not only are the functions of narrative important but also the focus. Individuals centre their stories on the significant experiences in their lives rather than on routine events or on 'vacuous time' as Järvinen calls it (p. 58). The latter seem to be irrelevant unless they are connected with that experience. For instance, a patient will tell the dramatic story of an illness, its process and treatment but only talk of routine events when they are disrupted or when normality cannot be achieved.

One of the effects of storytelling in research, though this is not always a stated or even intended goal, is to alleviate suffering and make people feel better. Pennebaker (2000) and Brody (2003), for instance, acknowledge that storytelling can perform a healing function. As stories are indexical, that is, they indicate real events and experiences, they help the individuals to create meaning and to master the experiences. Of course, remembering might also trigger ill effects but researchers should be prepared for these, and an ethical stance demands that people who suffer after telling their story in a research setting have counselling or other advice in place to manage these problems should they occur. In narrative research, specific ethical issues arise which will be discussed in Chapter 5.

Summary

This chapter has focused on narrative research, outlining its typologies, models and features. It has also described the differences between narrative and other forms of qualitative research. The importance of the functions of narrative inquiry has been highlighted. In the following chapter we shall narrow the focus to the use of narrative research in nursing.

3 Narrative Research in Nursing

Narrative, as a concept, has generated much interest in health-related disciplines and particularly in nursing, appealing to the profession because it functions so readily as a focus for anti-positivist analyses of nursing interventions (Freshwater, 2002). This makes it ripe for appropriation, and as such it is important that the meaning of narrative, and indeed related concepts (for example, story, plot, explanation, account), are adequately defined and delimited if they are to become genuine foci for nursing inquiry (Wiltshire, 1995; Frid et al., 2000; Freshwater and Rolfe, 2004). These concepts were described and defined in Chapter 2, and we do not intend to revisit those aspects of narrative research in detail here except where they further expand our discussion of their application and utilisation in nursing research.

Within the nursing literature too the terms 'narrative' and 'story' are used interchangeably. Wiltshire (1995), over a decade ago, discussed the concept of story and narrative and its connection to explanation and account, arguing that story and narrative were different by virtue of the fact that they tend to imply a democracy of equals. He notes:

> It is helpful to make distinction between a verbal account of illness, produced in a dialogue with and elicited by a nurse and a narrative written and initiated by the patient in his or her own right. Therapeutic claims may be used in both forms but they are different, and this difference, as well as the therapeutic importance of narrative forms needs to be clarified (Wiltshire, 1995: 56).

It is interesting to reflect upon how and why narrative research has taken such a hold in nursing and health care. In this chapter we outline some of the background to its inclusion and how it has been used to develop nurse education and nursing practice, its significance in terms of nursing knowledge, nursing research and scholarship and reasons why it appears to fit within the caring–healing and holistic framework of nursing care. It is suggested that nursing has become more and more technical at the expense of the human qualities of empathy, love and compassion. Freshwater and Stickley (2003), arguing for the restoration of the value of love in therapeutic and caring relationships including nursing relationships, ask: 'What is nursing if it is not the provision of one human being caring for another?' Within the current climate of evidence based practice, managed care, clinical outcomes and national standards, the value of human relationships (which is not necessarily a measurable phenomenon) and the associated emotion and meaning are lost. Nurses, disillusioned by the loss of meaning and relationships in their everyday practices, have turned to a variety of alternatives to enable them to foster more intimate alliances (note, for example, the rise in complementary therapies). Narrative research also emphasises intimate alliances, working closely with the personal truths and core values of both the researcher and the participant. In this sense narrative research attempts to rehabilitate the person, restoring the experiencing person to the centre of inquiry, and is akin to a humanistic and holistic approach to patient care; that is to say that narrative research can be described as person centred, as are many nursing models and theories (for example those of Margaret Newman, Martha Rogers, Jean Watson and Anne Boykin). This does not mean, however, that narrative research is self-centred; it is quite different (see details in Chapter 4). Moreover, representations of narrative research seek to repopulate the text, locating not only the participants but also the researcher firmly in the process.

The rise of narrative research in nursing

It is fair to say that the narrative turn in social science has had a significant and lasting impact on approaches to research in nursing. However, the use of narrative research in both nursing inquiry and nurse education is not new and does indeed have its own history. There are many factors which have influenced the increasing and at times overwhelming interest in narrative research across nursing and allied health professionals. Whilst we cannot attend to all of them in this chapter, we briefly examine those that we perceive have had significant and lasting effects. These include:

- Lack of relevance of research findings to clinical practice
- Backlash against the dominant discourse of evidence based practice
- A move beyond the subject–object divide
- Disillusionment with dehumanising care
- The drive for inclusiveness represented in the user/carer involvement movement
- Quest for an approach that values the therapeutic relationship at the heart of nursing

- Emphasis on reflective practice
- Appreciation of both the art and science of nursing
- Desire to explicate the quintessence of care through research
- The search for meaning in suffering

Frid et al. (2000) argue that narratives are presented both as a method of nursing research and as a way of presenting (improved) knowledge about nursing care. In their discussion they suggest that the term 'narrative' first appeared in the nursing literature in 1997 (they use CINAHL (Cumulative Index to Nursing and Allied Health Literature) as a marker of this). Hence, narrative, as cited in the nursing indices, is entering its 10th anniversary, meaning that, in this context at least, it is still a relatively young and innovative method. Interestingly, it is fair to assume that narrative research in nursing was published and available prior to this date, but perhaps struggled to be accepted in the indexed journals. Authors committed to the concept of caring in nursing were developing narrative inquiry earlier than 1997; see, for example, Bartol (1989), Boykin and Schoenhofer (1990), Sandelowski (1991), Vezeau (1993, 1994) and Maeve (1994). Such writers consider narrative to be fundamental, central and implicit to the nature, structure and indeed explication and expression of both nursing care and nursing knowledge (which are inextricably linked).

We begin by discussing the relevance and application of evidence based practice in nursing and the impact of this on clinical practice, practice improvement and nursing knowledge.

Evidence based practice and clinical relevance

Many authors have expressed their concern about the apparent lack of impact that nursing research has made on practice (Bircumshaw, 1990; Le May et al., 1998; Rolfe et al., 2001; Bishop and Freshwater, 2003). Over 20 years ago Sheehan (1986) asserted that applying research findings in nursing practice was perhaps the biggest challenge facing nursing research. Walsh and Ford (1989), for example, confronted the myth and ritual surrounding nursing practice, arguing that nurses behaved in certain ways because they had always behaved in this way. Prior to this, Greenwood (1984) rationalised that nurses, because of a lack of knowledge and a lack of belief regarding the findings, did not use research. She added that often nurses did not see the research findings as relevant to their practice because in fact they were not always relevant.

Nurses and nurse academics, like other health professionals, have been caught up in the paradigm wars, rehearsing the relative merits and limitations of quantitative and qualitative methodologies, both of which evoke criticisms of their epistemological bases. Whilst being actively engaged in the debate about the epistemological and the methodological credibility of research approaches to nursing was and continues to be an inevitable part of the process, it would seem that the debate itself has become limiting. The researcher is apt to get polarised into an either/or position, rather than seeing an alternative beyond the two opposing approaches. In the heat of the debate a power struggle ensues, each researcher seeing their own paradigm as the 'right' one for the job. And although the power relationships between the participant and researcher differ in each methodological approach, they are nevertheless inherent within the research process itself and as such are inescapable. Mixed methods research has also generated a great deal of interest amongst nurse researchers of late. Certainly, the discourse of mixed methods research has become more visible in recent years, as evidenced in the proliferation of research texts, papers, dedicated conferences and special editions of journals (Freshwater, 2006). Bryman (2006) suggests that there is a need to evaluate the current state of play with regard to mixed methods research, to take stock as it were, both across and within disciplines. Hence, even this apparent move to integrate methodology is not without its problems and critiques and of course has its own narrative.

Josselson and Lieblich (2001) argue that to date narrative approaches have avoided becoming paradigmatic in terms of method, although this does not mean that narrative research has been free from criticism or has avoided being caught up in the debate. Most recently the debate, at least in nursing and the allied health professions, has focused on the concept of evidence, more specifically evidence based practice. Nursing commentators have questioned the applicability in particular of the evidence based *medicine* movement to all disciplines within the health care team (Kitson, 1997; Salvage, 1998; Freshwater and Rolfe, 2004). Kitson (1997: 34), for example, remarks: 'It is not sufficient to change the name to evidence based practice or evidence based health-care without considering the impact on the conceptual framework upon which it is being built.'

French (1999) concurs with Kitson (1997), suggesting that evidence based medicine, not necessarily as it was conceived but as it has been interpreted, may have had a deleterious effect on the development of nursing and health care. He provides three arguments in support of this conclusion:

- Evidence based medicine further medicalises the environment within which health care is operationalised.
- Evidence based medicine emphasises the value of positivist research, defining evidence in purely quantitative forms.

- Evidence based medicine pays little attention to the practitioner's understanding of the situation and as such propositional knowledge.

We would further these arguments, and contend that this particular conceptualisation of evidence based medicine also potentially disregards personal and aesthetic knowledge, what might be termed situated and intuitive wisdom (Polanyi, 1962; Carper, 1978; Chinn and Watson, 1994; Freshwater, 1998, 2004) – domains of knowledge which are all too frequently missed or trivialised within the scientific discourse of healthcare. This is an argument that Hunter (1996), a professor of literature with strong involvement in medical education, concurs with. She admits to being baffled by the medical profession's preoccupation with the gold standard of randomised controlled trials in clinical practice, espousing that medicine is better distinguished as moral, interpretative, narrative knowing which relies heavily on practical reasoning (Hunter, 1996). Greenhalgh and Hurwitz (1998) have done much to validate this perspective amongst medical colleagues. We do not wish to reject evidence of best practice based on quantitative and experimental methods, nor is this chapter about to turn into another quantitative/qualitative debate. We do, though, want to challenge the applicability of the hierarchy of evidence model and its preferred research methods to all nursing practice and to encourage nurses and other health professionals to approach all research, as they do practice, with reflection, deliberation and therefore informed intention and critique. This of course includes narrative.

What is evidence based practice?

Nursing has traditionally worked towards improving patient care and outcomes by using scientific evidence and therein evidence based practice (McClarey and Duff, 1997). Defined as the process of systematically reviewing, appraising and using contemporaneous research findings as the basis for clinical decisions (Rosenberg and Donald, 1995; Kitson, 1997), evidence based practice is clearly linked to patient care. Nevertheless, it also needs to be acknowledged that patient care and therefore patient outcomes are contextual. As such, evidence based practice needs to be contextualised within both the practitioners' and the patients' local experience. Nursing is often based on individual judgement which is made within a particular context (Sandelowski, 1991), a context that can be made explicit in terms of its impact and influence through narrative. Evidence based practice demands that nursing maintains a closer compatibility between caring beliefs and caring actions.

Naturally there is some discrepancy across the disciplines as to what constitutes evidence. The traditional approach to examining evidence acts as if all evidence were external to the practitioner with little recognition of the body of evidence that nurses carry around with them (Benner, 1984). A number of writers have attempted to respond to this question (Freshwater, 1998; Rolfe, 1998; Bonnell, 1999; Closs and Cheater, 1999; Colyer and Kamath, 1999; Freshwater and Rolfe, 2004). Harvey et al. (1997) describe the varieties of evidence available for decision making as a continuum which is usually unequally weighted towards evidence in practice derived from randomised controlled trials (RCTs). This is also true of the many research and development strategies informed by the hierarchy of evidence model (Canadian Task Force on the Periodic Health Examination, 1979; Long, 1998) in which the quality of evidence is assessed in terms of its level (McClarey and Duff, 1997). The highest level of evidence seen within this model (level 1) is that which is obtained from at least one properly designed RCT, with opinions of respected authorities, clinical experience and descriptive studies having much less credibility (level 5). There is little doubt that when clinical practice raises questions about the impact a form of care has on patients, randomised controlled trials are a useful way of providing answers. Many nurses, however, feel uncomfortable with the idea of RCTs in nursing (Seers and Milne, 1997), which do not always capture knowledge based in relationality, aesthetic experience and intuition. In addition Marks-Maran (1999: 9) contends that evidence available for making nursing decisions 'will not be found in any randomised controlled trial because that is not the appropriate methodology for research into nursing'. It is posited here that this, in part, is due to the perception that RCTs reduce the care-giving experience to small parts, with little attention being given to the whole (Seers and Milne, 1997). Some practitioners have adopted quality of life measures in order to reflect a holistic approach to researching clinical practice, but unfortunately almost all quality of life measures involve a reduction of quality into quantity and the imposition of one personal set of values on to those of the other (Hopkins, 1992; Greenhalgh and Hurwitz, 1998).

It would be easy to attribute the developments and innovations in nursing research to the ongoing disillusionment with traditional approaches to practice and articulating research and the resulting lack of application of (relevant) findings. However, the emerging trends in research methods in nursing have a narrative of their own, and of course a relationship to time and space. Changes in nursing research also occur within a bigger context, one in which the preoccupation with logical positivism is gradually losing its foothold. That is to say that approaches to research in nursing need to be viewed in context, a context that has, until recent years, favoured method over meaning resulting, at times, in 'obscure trivial investigations that idealize statistical procedures but stray far from concern with the people being studied' (Josselson and Lieblich, 2001: 278). The drive to find ways of making research findings relevant, readable, interesting and transferable is not insignificant in its impact on methodology; for methods and modes of representation are inextricably linked. It is predominantly, although not exclusively, qualitative methods that seek novel, meaningful and transferable representational styles. Narrative inquiry, and representation of the same, take one step closer to the edge, in that they encourage the voice of the researcher and the participants (whoever they are) and their contextual relationship to be prioritised (and its historical, social, ethical and political base).

In the age of managed care, success is measured by efficiency and cost reduction. Whilst legislators use the language of care, what appears to matter most to those in power is the efficiency of productivity. 'In the process of McDonaldising the nursing profession, there is a danger of inviting the notion of care – the very act upon which the profession is established – to leave the room' (Freshwater and Stickley, 2003: p. 00). Any of us who have been on the receiving end of hospital care know only too well the demoralising effects of treatment without care. Similarly, we recognise and appreciate the treatment with care that makes the experience of being a patient all the more bearable. Without care people are treated as objects, meaning is lost, and we become victims of a dehumanising system as we seek out the smile and care from the nurse/professional who attends to us. The art of nursing is not only rendered invisible; it withers and deforms.

Holistic care versus dehumanised care

The debate surrounding the notion of holism and its relationship to the art of nursing is as well rehearsed as the deliberations around the quantitative–qualitative dichotomy in the research arena. Nursing is much more than the application of quantitative and experimental research findings (Johnson, 1994). In order to develop this argument further it is helpful to refer back to the well used definitive work of Barbara Carper. In her seminal article Carper (1978) identified four fundamental patterns of knowing in nursing: empirics, aesthetics, personal knowledge and ethical knowledge. Despite Carper's work being described as one of the greatest contributions to the understanding of nursing (Chinn and Kramer, 1995; Silva et al., 1995), nursing still struggles to apportion equal attention to two of Carper's ways of knowing, namely the aesthetic and the personal. The four patterns of knowing are seen as complementary, with their integration leading to a rich understanding of the discipline of nursing (Bird, 1994). Whilst Carper (1978) herself did not formulate the ways of knowing into a hierarchical model, traditional modernist approaches to research have the tendency to do so, as in the hierarchical model of evidence. The most alarming feature of the hierarchy of evidence model is its apparent lack of respect for qualitative research and for aesthetic and personal ways of knowing which, when applied to nursing, depotentiates and to some extent invalidates the knowledge embedded in the art of nursing and implicitly the knowledge derived from narrative.

The art of nursing

The art of nursing is a familiar concept and refers to the personal wisdom and insight that the individual care-giver develops along the route (Katims, 1993; Marks-Maran, 1999). It is generally thought of as knowledge that is not grounded in science or theory but is rather the intuitive application of formal knowledge (Katims, 1993). Nursing as an aesthetic experience is a lived experience, manifest as one's actions and one's interactions with the world. This is always lived by the author. Hence, nursing when viewed as aesthetic experience transforms the nurse from observer to participant (Begley, 1996), and who would argue that nursing is not a participatory experience? The philosophical connections between practice experience and aesthetics can be traced back to Aristotle who used the term 'praxis' to describe the integration of senses, thought, action and meaning. Derived from the Greek, 'praxis' literally means 'I do' and relates to the execution of a job well done (Labkowicz, 1967). But how does one judge whether a job is well done? As previously indicated, evidence based practice, as derived from medicine, usually applies some external measure or standard as the judge. Thus excellence in performance is marked by some external factor, rather than being viewed as an internal demand that the nurse strives for and which requires both nurturing and sustaining (Katims, 1993). From this latter perspective nurse care-giving becomes an end in itself as opposed to nursing activities being directed towards an end that is different from the process of care-giving. Nurse care-giving is both the art and the science. Narrative is also an end in itself, one that examines the process and product of nursing, suffering and caring in a meaningful way.

The use of narratives encourages the researcher/practitioner not only to consider individuals as unique but also to promote caring for the whole person rather than having a fragmented view which concentrates on a symptom or disease (Capasso, 1998; Freshwater and Stickley, 2003; Freshwater, 2004). Further nursing narratives are open to multiple interpretations, allowing wider professional issues from a variety of perspectives to be explored within the profession (Lupton, 1994), including that of meaning, purpose and intention.

Meaningful nursing inquiry

When questioning the purpose of research, Braud (1994) argues that there are three motivations:

- To learn about the world and other people in order to predict and control
- To understand the world in the service of curiosity and wonder
- To appreciate the world and delight in its myriad of entities

The first motivation for research is instrumental and has a utilitarian value. Knowledge is seen as power and the researcher enlists large and random samples in order to generate general principles. This motivation is in complete contrast to the second and third, which appear to have more in common. The second motivation for research views the world as a puzzle and seeks to understand how the puzzle fits together, whilst the third motivation is based on variety, discovery and surprise. Research emanating from current research appears to originate, in the main, from the first motivation, with perhaps some influence from the second. Research that is motivated by variety, discovery and surprise requires the capacity to tolerate uncertainty, something that is not alien to nurses and results in evidence of good practice as presented in a detailed map of some new territory or the revelation of some previously unknown paths in old territory: what might be called the extraordinary, manifest in the ordinary.

Research that is motivated by the need to understand and appreciate the world of practice and caring is much more likely to originate in Braud's (1994) third motivation, and to re-present its findings using aesthetic expressions that are narrative, poetry, literature and art, all of which incidentally involve cognitions. Thus, the nurse researcher who embraces the aesthetic dimension can be seen as an integral inquirer, one who uses a pluralistic epistemology, pooling all aspects of the self including bodily reactions, emotions, feelings, intuitions, cognitions and aesthetic sensibilities (Braud, 1994).

We have pondered over where this type of evidence fits into the hierarchy of evidence model that currently informs the definition of 'best evidence'. It could be argued that this type of research fits, if anywhere, into the third category, that is, alongside clinical experience, thus placing aesthetic and personal practical knowledge in an inferior position and therein perpetuating the theory–practice gap. Once again nursing research potentially finds itself in a marginalised position and, as Sandelowski (1991: 164) states, remains caught in the 'inherently contradictory project of making something scientific out of everything biographical'. Instead nursing needs to establish an understanding of evidence based practice that is congruent with its emerging paradigm (Marks-Maran, 1999). Narrative and the aesthetic dimension of caring are integral to pluralistic inquiry which incorporates all sensibilities. The hierarchy of evidence as it currently stands allows little room for the patient's perspective in the research process. How often, when conducting a systematic review of the literature, does the researcher come across autobiographical illness narratives and accounts of 'evidence based care' from the patient's vantage point? How many patients are involved in (and realistically could be involved in) the collection and analysis of data generated from a randomised controlled trial? This is an important consideration in view of the move towards consumer 'involvement' in the research process, as opposed to being 'subjects' of the research process (NHSE, 1998). The user involvement movement has clearly affected both the conduct and process of research in healthcare as users and carers become involved at all stages of the inquiry, including that of commissioning and determining appropriate methods. We turn now to the relationship between user involvement and narrative research.

User involvement and narrative research

The notion of agency is one of the most highly valued terms in social science, often used in contrast to the term 'victim' to describe the level of power and autonomy ascribed to an individual within a specified context (Nielsen, 1999). Within contemporary healthcare discourse, the notion of agency is being explored and developed from a variety of perspectives, increasingly through involving the users of healthcare facilities in decision-making processes. This is also true of consumer involvement in nursing, nurse education and nursing research. Critiques of modern medicine comment on the overemphasis of healthcare policy on service rather than on the users of those services, thus marginalising the voices of those users and carers accessing the service (DHSS, 1983). Recent White Papers in the UK and across other westernised countries address these criticisms, talking in terms of partnerships and lay participation in service delivery, research and education (DH, 1998, 2000). It is essential, then, that a variety of research approaches are utilised in order to ensure not only that questions are answered, but also that multiple voices can be heard, including those of the user. The narrative voice, rather like the user's voice, has been marginalised in the past. Despite the current emphasis on inquiry using narrative approaches, it is important that such processes be used appropriately and that they be relevant to the research questions, otherwise it too can become a tokenistic venture.

Every profession has a standard story that is constructed for the constraints of practice and practitioners and their everyday work. One such standard story is that of empowerment and the sharing of re-sponsibility with the patient and their carers. Whilst there is a growing expectation within Government that the NHS should involve users and the public to a greater extent in decision making, healthcare discourse often fails to consider the voice of the patient in the therapeutic encounter. The need to involve service users more actively in health-care research is a natural progression to establish a genuine two-way relationship between health science researchers, health providers and users (Wood and Wilson Barnett, 1999). Involving users in research, education and practice developments, and listening to the narratives of these experiences in particular, can be both empowering and valid-ating for the patient and is one way of influencing inequalities in the patient/professional relationship.

Social, psychological and physical elements are recognised as pivotal dimensions in the structure of human services, and as such professionals need to be aware of the types of structures, the underpinning values that drive them and ways that they can be expressed. Hughson and Brown (1988) provide some examples of beliefs that are recognised as fundamental to the practice of professionals in relation to consumers in human services, namely:

- Self-determination
- Protection of civil and human rights
- Individualisation
- Acknowledgements of humanity

The use of patient narratives as an approach to research, education and practice allows students and practitioners to listen to patients' experi-ences and consider the viewpoint and understanding of the patient/client and their informal carers' needs, as opposed to a professional's definition of need (Wood and Wilson Barnett, 1999). Working in partnership with carers/service users requires all participants to acknowledge the tensions that exist between the nurse's duty of care and the service user's right to self-determination. By meaningful involvement in the research experience, all participants can explore issues of paternalism and empowerment, gaining insight into the different perspectives. This deeper insight can assist the practitioner to look at the complex area of power relationships and allows the practitioner/

researcher/student to practise their interpersonal skills, developing democratic ways of working with people in their care within a supportive environment.

Narratives in nursing research: beyond dualism?

Over decades of debate the ambiguous stance that researchers have carried towards the objective–subjective divide has been scrutinised, interrogated and examined in minute detail. In 1994 Vezeau asked: 'How can nursing develop knowledge about persons in health and transition that acknowledges that ambiguity?' She answers her own question, referring to the use of creative narrative as aesthetic inquiry.

What can narrative research offer the nursing profession?

The use of narratives enables the world of the patient to be explored, allowing the person to explain the many facets of their personality and values and their experience of the professional–patient relationship. The patient is central to nursing and healthcare; it could be argued therefore that a forum to listen and understand the world of the patient is paramount to nursing knowledge (Repper, 2000). Frid et al. (2000) outline a number of applications and benefits of narrative for both nursing research and nursing care, stating that:

> 'The narrative creates an innovative imitation of something that previously occurred by imitating the practical action (praxis). However, the narration does not function as repetition – it creates a new reformulated description. The narrative is thereby able to cast new light on that which has previously been experienced as familiar' (Frid et al., 2000: 697).

Freshwater links narrative with reflection and reflexivity, similarly arguing that narrative, like reflection, casts new light through the rich interplay of insight, foresight and hindsight in constructive and deconstructive processes. Vezeau (1994: 42) also linked reflection to narrative as she says 'Readers bring reflection and openness in allowing the "shock of recognition".' She goes on: 'In this process, narrative demonstrates a profound weaving of human context and responses that provide a solid base for knowledge development in nursing.'

We further suggest that the narrative inquiry:

- Makes nursing work visible
- Attends to all types of knowledge including the personal and aesthetic dimensions
- Influences practice through developing local and contingent knowledge
- Provides meaning for routinised practices that can seem ritualistic and meaningless
- Facilitates interprofessional understanding of clinical situations
- Enables patients and narrators to derive meaning from their illness experience
- Facilitates and fosters creative thinking, blending artistry and craft with theoretical knowing
- Creates a therapeutic milieu in which narrators and listeners can be transformed
- Allows multiple voices and multiple perspectives to co-exist
- Makes clinical reasoning processes explicit

The dynamics of narrative also enable the participant and researcher to have a multidimensional voice, allowing the many facets of an experience to be intertwined, giving the listener a greater understanding. A story, if recreated, will not be the same because no two encounters are identical, but it (the narrative) considers lived experiences which are grounded in reality to describe the process or plot. Narratives also allow both the listener and the narrator to reflect and consider how the story influences the present. Earlier we mentioned Carper's different ways of knowing. Storytelling is also a way of knowing (Abma, 1999). It is suggested that when a story is narrated the teller is involved in the subject matter; it is part of their life experiences, a part of their identity. Researchers relate to the narrator and the story at the same time. There is no distancing from the reality, which may occur if a third party later told the story (Brykczynska, 1997). Observation such as this, combined with theoretical and practical knowledge, assists in informing the choices about how to proceed in providing care.

The experience of illness

Understanding the illness experience is seen by many authors as vital to the caring role (Kleinman, 1988; Frank, 2000). Equally, it is important for the nurse to understand the experience of illness, for without this opportunity to reflect, the nurse may not be conscious of the issues and the importance of 'being with' the patient (Capasso, 1998). Communication and understanding a different perspective may not be experienced and in practice may leave a patient feeling isolated and alone in their illness (Newman, 1994). As Vezeau (1994: 46), who describes narrative as active inquiry, suggests, it possesses healing properties, not unlike the work of Arthur Frank, noting that narratives help people to make sense of their world and live in it 'as participants and not combatants'. Living in the world of others also means finding creative ways of entering and experiencing that world.

Narrative and creativity

The humanities are a collection of liberal arts, their main purpose being to broaden an individual's outlook on human life and the context and values in which it is lived (Brykczynska, 1997). This allows the individual (in this case the nurse) to consider perspectives and alternative methods of expression. The use of illness narratives in this way can help understanding and provide an explanation or an appreciation, which can promote the importance of interpersonal care (Styles and Moccia, 1993). In addition to language, the creative arts (Jonas, 1994; Watson and Chinn, 1994; Predeger, 1996; Picard, 2000) have been used as a medium to express or explore lived experience or feelings of illness.

The use of creative literature in clinical education and practice has been reported by nurses, medics and therapists as an aid to helping patients; as a way of seeing the whole patient (Younger, 1990); as a way of fostering compassion (Young-Mason, 1988); and more recently as a way of accessing evidence based practice (Greenhalgh and Hurwitz, 1998). A brief literature review revealed a small number of articles that describe practical engagement with the creative arts, 'practical engagement' meaning situations where practitioners or clients express themselves through a variety of arts media to explore and discover personal truth, insight and meaning about particular life experiences. These experiences may lie more within the personal or professional sense of self, or most likely embrace both. The literature reviewed fell within three broad areas of application: healing, education and research. For the most part, the literature on the creative arts is multidimensional and incorporates healing, educational and research based elements, though one aspect is often more strongly featured than others. In the literature the variety of creative processes referred to includes: narrative, imaginal storytelling (through the use of metaphor), dream work, poetry, collage, drawing and painting, drama, movement and music, photography, sculpture, and the creation of fabric based artefact.

Narratives in research are increasingly used not only to collect data (Rittman et al., 1997), which can be analysed using traditional qualitative techniques and other contemporary data analysis frames (see Chapter 8) but also as a way of teaching and learning and a way of creating meaning in suffering. Narratives also allow the practitioner, the student and other professionals to listen to the experiences of the person, to understand suffering or confusion and help the carer to gain an insight into what Newman (1999) describes as a 'tolerance for uncertainty'. A nurse may not 'know' but must be accepting and be present if therapeutic relationships are to be maintained. In this sense narratives are one factor that has helped nurses decide how best to approach individualised care and to achieve a sense of the bigger picture.

Narrative in nurse education

The dominance of the medical model in nursing, traditionally associated with the nurse as expert and a task oriented approach to care, is now making way to a more patient centred approach and to seamless continuity of care. The user involvement movement, the move towards community care, the emphasis on health promotion and the changing role of the carer in caring for their relatives at home have all impacted on the view of the expert. Increasingly the patient/carer is seen as the expert and as possessing clinical knowledge. In other words patients are recognised as being the experts in their own condition, and/or carers often know the most appropriate form of treatment (see Freshwater, 2002). Views of nursing have changed, and nurse education has had to make some pretty radical shifts – and of course so has research.

Freshwater and Stickley (2003) note that narrative is an important part of an emotionally intelligent curriculum. Lindsay and Smith (2003: 121) argue for a research based narrative curriculum in nursing education. Further they contend that narrative 'matters to construction of nursing praxis and to life long learning as a nurse'. They refer to the 'dominant narratives of the medical model for patient care and corporate language and practices in health care institutions'. Moreover clinical reasoning involves making sense of and deriving meaning from knowledge gathered from encounters with patients. Observations, combined with theoretical and practice knowledge, inform the choices made about how to proceed in care.

Summary

Greenhalgh and Hurwitz (1998: 251) contend that narrative moves away from the reification of generalisable truths, asking 'How then, can we square the circle of upholding individual narrative in a world where valid and generalisable truths are population-derived evidence?'

Over recent years, nurses and nurse researchers have been working to separate narrative as a data collection method and narrative as a methodology in itself. Narrative research presents nursing and nursing research with a substantial challenge, that is, to step beyond the prevailing modernist notion of what counts as evidence and to seek different answers to the human situation. Marks-Maran (1999) suggests that a postmodernist view of evidence of best practice in nursing would not only include evidence from both qualitative and quantitative research but would also draw upon the values of patients and nurses, and upon intuitive and experiential knowledge. We argue that a recent marker of the turn away from the modernist notion of evidence is the development of a literary consciousness through the impulse to narrate. Narrative is just one source of aesthetic knowing in nursing and there are many more methods of aesthetic expressions under investigation. In the context of narrative 'the concept of truth is reclaimed from logical positivism' and is 'distinguished from other kinds of formal science truths by its emphasis on the life-like intelligible and plausible story' (Sandelowski, 1991: 164).

The contribution of the narrative approach to nursing, medicine and allied professions' knowledge and practice is now reasonably well documented (see for example Jones, 1990; Younger, 1990; Darbyshire, 1995; Greenhalgh and Hurwitz, 1998; Charmaz, 1999; Aranda and Street, 2000; Hurwitz et al., 2004). However, owing (in part) to the overemphasis of the traditional medical model of professional practice and scientific approaches to research, narrative methods in nursing research have paradoxically been underused and undervalued and, to some extent, continue to be poorly understood in terms of their contribution to identifying and sharing good practice and partnerships in care (Darbyshire, 1995; Savage, 2000). This is paradoxical also because narrative research has simultaneously been adopted by nurses who appear to be enamoured with narrative as a form of inquiry, yet do not necessarily understand it in its/their own historical, political and ethical context. The remainder of this text is dedicated to explicating and drilling down into narrative research, within the context of nursing and the allied professions. Our aim is to provide a practical, theoretical and philosophical basis for conducting high quality, rigorous and credible narrative inquiry.

4 Narrative and the Construction of Identity

One assertion commonly found in the literature around narrative is that the stories people tell to and about themselves also, in some way, construct who they are. Such assertions have not gone unchallenged; in fact the distinction between the narrating subject and the subject of narration is the topic of a complex and ongoing ontological debate (Cohan and Shires, 1988; Butler, 1993; Rose, 1996; Redman, 2005). Whatever perspective is taken, identity and knowledge are viewed as inextricably linked and in a seamless relationship with social and personal practices; identity is also linked to the notion of selfhood, agency and power.

Redman (2005), in his analysis of the narrative formation of identity, questions the extent to which individual identities are fabricated by and in narratives as opposed to having inherent capacities that precede any identity building that narrative might do. The literature presents competing ways of theorising the relationship between narrative and identity formation. Writers examine, on the one hand, the degree to which people are spoken by narratives (i.e. created by and in narratives) and on the other hand the degree to which we, as individuals, speak narratives. Or, put another way, whether we are invented by our social context or alternatively whether we construct/invent our social context. Of course it is not necessarily the case that we are *either* narrated *or* narrating; in fact we can and do have the experience of both. Both positions hold some attraction and are seductive, with the potential for *suture* which will be described in more depth at a later point. In this chapter we briefly explore the complex ontological concepts of the self, social construction, identity and identity formation, and these in relation to narrative, the narrating subject and the subject of narrative. We begin with the much disputed concept of the self.

Selfhood and the search for identity

The debate surrounding the nature of and indeed the existence of the self has been the subject of many philosophical and theoretical dialogues. Freshwater (2002: 1) notes that the concept of the self has been variously described in psychological terms, modernist terms, spiritual terms, biological terms, sociological terms and latterly postmodernist terms. These recent discussions challenge not only the permanence but also the presence of a self at all. Such theoretical debates can loosely be divided into two camps, those related to ego theories and those related to bundle theories (for a comprehensive review of these perspectives see Gallagher and Shear (1999), Blackmore (2001) and Freshwater (2002)). Proponents of ego theories believe in the existence of a persistent self, whereas bundle theorists deny any such thing. Rather like the postmodernist view, the apparent unified self is viewed as a collection of ever changing experiences (bundles) that are tied together through a number of means, including narrative. Thus the dominant modernist view of the self as rational, finite, self-motivated and predictable across time and contexts is compared in more recent constructivist literature with a conversational resource, in which the self is viewed as a story we tell ourselves and others. Elliott (2005), for example, refers to this distinction as being the difference between a self that has a stable set of characteristics and dispositions and a reflexive self. From this latter perspective, the self is equal to: 'a continuous construction of self-narrative, aiming to secure a sense of historical continuity, directionality and coherence among what often appear to be loosely connected "selves" that may seem to act differently depending on the circumstances' (Androutsopoulou, 2001: 282). This highlights the difference between an open, situational and discursively sensitive human subjectivity, as opposed to subjectivity based on depth psychological issues contingent upon early identification and ego development.

This problematising of the self as being iterative, interactive and contextually dependent clearly has implications not only for identity formation, but importantly, in the context of this book, for our understanding and application of narrative inquiry, not least in that it challenges dearly held beliefs that the self can be observed, diagnosed and improved. For a dynamic and reflexive identity cannot ever be fully known in any real and 'truthful' way. As Elliott (2005: 124) notes:

> 'Individuals cannot be understood as having a fixed identity that is ontologically prior to their position in the social world. Identity is not to be found inside a person (like a kernel with a nut shell) but rather it is relational and inheres in the interactions a person has with each other.'

This also, of course, impacts on the way in which the self of the researcher is used in the research process (we come to this in Chapter 13).

Cobley (2004) views the self as key to narrative concerns, which he sees as being related to identity. Referring to Gergen and Gergen (1988: 37), he notes: 'It is fairly well known in the modern world that social circumstances, and the existence of the self within them, are to a large extent socially constructed by texts and the narratives they frequently contain.' Cobley (2004: 234), again, defines identity as 'The perception and feeling of belonging to a particular group as a result of commonalities of experience, status and physical existence.' Such commonalities, he suggests, 'can revolve around social class, gender, sexuality, class, age, occupation, ethnicity, nationality and so on. Identity can also derive from the experiences of much more local phenomena such as individual or familial circumstances.' In his writings Cobley (2004) provides many examples of ways in which the self and identity are central to the narrative endeavour, describing one of the greatest ever narratives, Honer's *Odyssey*, as a story of identity and a voyage to the self. The term 'identity' can be understood in a number of different ways. Elliott (2005) speaks of two, both drawn from Latin: *idem* meaning identical, the same, or continuity, and *ipse* meaning permanence through time without sameness and self-same (both of course are linked to temporality but have a different relationship to the same). Like most authors we prefer to avoid a polarisation between essentialist and constructionist views of the self, allowing both to coexist and comment on our life experience. Like Gergen and Gergen (1988), we believe that the self is both stable and dynamic, and that the push and pull of opposing forces lead to both change and continuity.

Bruner (1991) observes that self is the common coin of our speech. There is no such thing as a self waiting to be revealed or discovered: rather a self is constructing and reconstructing, is dynamic and ongoing in relation to context. Self making, then, according to Bruner, is a narrative art, an internal and external activity, and principally a means of establishing our uniqueness. Telling others about oneself, however, is more complex than just making up a story about oneself and telling it to another. As Bruner notes, it depends on what: 'we (I) think they (I) think we ought to be like – or what selves in general ought to be like' (p. 84). Who then is really telling the story; which aspect of the self, if it exists, is foreground? Psychoanalytic and psychological literature has grappled with these issues for decades, identifying true and false self systems, self-concepts, organismic selves and divided selves, personas and mask wearers.

Putting on a face or wearing a mask is an issue that is related to narrative, specifically in regard to rigour and trustworthiness of the data, i.e. are the data made up? Speaking of the improvisational narrative which Holstein and Gubrium (1995: 28) suggest 'combines aspects of experience, emotion, opinion, and expectation, connecting disparate parts into a coherent, meaningful whole, the respondent does not just "make things up" in the sense that he or she is "true to life" – faithful to subjectively meaningful experience – even as it is creatively, spontaneously rendered'. We relate this to the development of an ethical and moral self, which will not be addressed here in any detail; nevertheless, we do come back to this in Chapter 5.

According to Elliott (2005: 124): 'Postmodern scepticism about the existence of an unproblematic, unified and coherent self has also opened up new possibilities for qualitative research to focus on the everyday practices by which individuals constantly construct and reconstruct their sense of individual identity.' Thus not only do contemporary views of the self, identity and identity formation provide an opportunity for narratologists to engage in novel, creative and dynamic research, but also, one could argue, the view of the self has been transformed over the years through the process of narrative.

We understand narrative research to be an interactive process in which the self is constructed, deconstructed and reconstructed through and by the telling of the narrative. Nevertheless, despite the close examination of the self, the end result is not a fixed identity; rather it is the new starting point. The search for an adequate sense of identity is a highly charged, emotional and potentially driven process (Freshwater and Robertson, 2002). Narrative does not reveal universal features of humankind but can be used to represent cultural difference and hybridity (Cobley, 2004). Hybridity pertains here to the way in which cultures (and individuals in cultures) construct narratives about themselves, editing out alien features of other cultures (subcultures/ individuals), positioning themselves in relation to others through difference and similarity.

So far we have been using the terms construction, deconstruction and social construction in relation to our debate surrounding the existence or not of a narrating self. It might be useful at this point to clarify what is meant when we use the term social construction and related terms. Social constructionism is principally concerned with explaining the influences upon and the processes by which people come to describe, explain, and account for the world in which they live (Daymon and Holloway, 2002). It attempts to articulate common forms of understanding as they are now, as they were in the past and as they might potentially develop in the future, linking the past, present and future through temporality (see Gergen and Gergen, 2003). Social constructionist inquiry thus focuses on multiple realities and relationships. At the centre of constructionist research is the reconstruction of stories around experiences (Gergen and Gergen, 2003).

The active self: identity in the wider context

Narrative, whilst focusing on the subjective experience of narrators, also takes into account the bigger picture by exploring wider societal and cultural experiences. Narrative is in fact a social activity, a product of interaction between cultural discourses, material circumstances and experience. Narrative then is not only bound up with individual identity formation but is also connected to large-scale identities such as nations, cultures and subcultures. Interestingly narrative is a common vehicle for transmitting those common identities to other nations, cultures and subcultures. Anderson (1991) rather nicely suggests that narrative helps to bind individuals in a nation through the concept of a 'meanwhile'. However, whilst cultural resources may provide guidelines to help individuals recount stories, they cannot determine the content of each individual narrative, rather 'the constructionist invitation is first to open the door to multiple traditions, each with their own particular view of knowledge and methodology' (Gergen and Gergen, 2003: 60).

Porter Abbott's (2002) rather extreme position is not only that narratives are a way of knowing ourselves but also that we can only know ourselves in so far as we are narrativised: 'it is through narrative that we know ourselves as active entities that operate through time' (2002: 123). Many authors view the principal component of story as character and action. Cobley (2004), for instance, points out that narrative has basic features, these being characters and situations. However, whilst many authors agree on this, a cautionary note should be added here, as commonly agreed features can sometimes lead to the temptation to standardise or universalise a process. Narrative research is certainly not about standardisation. Characters have agency, and can cause things to happen. Further, during action, characters reveal who they are, their motives and their strengths.

This notion of the character is significant in terms of our discussion about identity and self in narrative. Returning to our earlier comments about ego theories and bundle theories, one might begin to gain a sense of the impact of the researcher's starting point (i.e. beliefs and values regarding the self) and the way in which a self relates to the bigger world. In other words, the lens through which we understand the concept of self and identity will add a layer of complexity to the way in which characters are analysed and situated in the text. Forster (2005), for example, in his definitive work, *Aspects of the Novel*, describes flat and round characters; flat characters, he argues have no hidden complexity or depth and are rather predictable, lacking mystery. Round characters, in contrast, are more complex and not easily summed up, and seduce the reader into filling in the gaps.

Entering the social world

Characters can be seen to be engaged in the process of making an adjust-ment to or liberating from existing narratives as they flow between the internal world of the self and the external world of the other. Entering the social world is a lifetime's work; however, many ego theorists believe that the earliest life experiences are the most crucial in terms of iden-tity formation, although there are many identity crises throughout life.

The identity that is forming as the child enters the social world is a linguistically constrained identity. The problem with Freud's (1915) topographical model of the psyche was that it was primarily an inter-nal one with social pressures being channelled through a critical con-trolling superego. There is no room in this model for the creative co-regulation that characterises much social play. Education of feeling involves the refinement of sensibility through being opened up to poten-tialities and suffering from which the ego has shrunk. In facing the fear of ego death, the character is built up. Emotional change at this level brings with it psychic transformation through the imagination and leads to a greater flexibility of responses.

Ego theorists, for example, view the shift from attachment (and dependence) and merging to independence and separateness as stimu-lating an awakening to the interpersonal aspects of the self in the context of social and culturally embedded norms. The move away from mother into a world where emotions and needs are not mediated by one other, but by several others and a group, requires the individual to make an adaptation to the world and is a tumultuous journey. It is one that necessitates a separation not only of self from other, and the development of a relationship of self to other, but also a differenti-ation of needs and the discovery of our very essence. Sorting the seeds becomes a daily process of ruthless honesty that 'allows us grain by grain to discover our Being' (Woodman, 1985: 78). The process of sort-ing of the seeds leads to a differentiation of survival needs, sexual needs and higher order needs. But before the needs are differentiated, the indi-vidual can experience powerful emotions around injustice and fairness, often accepting their lot uncritically whilst simultaneously feeling themselves to be the victim. They may have a desire to contribute to life but fail to take responsibility for themselves. As the person's needs begin to differentiate, they are often plunged into an identity crisis. They are no longer who they were, and yet they are not yet who they are to become. It is at this stage of life that an individual can find him-self or herself changing careers, challenging existing relationships, developing a love of learning and experimenting, and not being able to stand still: experiencing both an avoidance of peace and also a search and maybe a longing for peace as the identity is forged.

Shifting identity: narratives as adjustment or liberation from self

Locating this discussion in the wider context of society, Rowan (2000) clearly articulates the difference between a narrative psychotherapy that seeks to help the client adjust, focusing on the removal of symptoms and enabling the client to return to 'normality', and liberation therapy. Liberation therapy, which is usually longer term than adjustment therapy, emphasises the underlying psycho-spiritual stage of development that is pushing for awareness through the symptoms being presented. Hence it has less well defined aims and as a result does not have clearly articulated outcomes.

So, whilst adjustment narrative might enable the client to accept the context of their lives and move within the current landscape, liberation narratives undermine the structural beliefs and emotions that underpin the problematic feelings. Persons are challenged to change the landscape they are in. Liberation narrative, then, may bring awareness of a whole new set of emotions, whose quality and tone are related to the whole (of the self) rather than the parts (subpersonalities), that is, they are more linked to existential angst than they are to neurotic anxiety.

In the various cycles of self development and identity formation, issues such as autonomy and responsibility, intimacy and solitude and the development of trust in the self become vitally important. There are analogous parallels in some research methods, specifically at the time of data collection and the writing of research dissertations, reports and papers, in which the deepening understanding of the data and the metaphorical birth of the findings can also be an emotionally demanding experience necessitating a high level of self-awareness and a reformulation of one's identity. These are often periods in the research in which the emotional heat is most strongly felt, both in the relationships with the participants and within oneself. In this sense it is a time during which awareness, authenticity and congruence of identity can be confronted. Thus, narrative research not only provides an opportunity to explore and examine the concept of identity formation and construction through personal narratives; it also provides an opportunity for researchers to reflect on their own experience of identity formation and reformation through the process of the inquiry itself. Of course, a degree of reflexivity and openness is required for this to take place.

As with all life experiences, conducting narrative research is a chance to learn something new about oneself and to engage in a transformatory process (Freshwater, 2000). The same opportunity is afforded the participants, as narrative research not only permits and encourages

participants to narrate themselves; it also facilitates the process of construction and reconstruction, creating space for renewal and closure
(Freshwater and Robertson, 2002), or, as Woodman (1985: 15) suggests,
opportunities to encounter both the known and the unknown aspects
of our identities: 'Birth is the death of the life we have known; death
is the birth of the life we have yet to live'. Redman (2005) seems to be
referring to this process of encountering ourselves and our situatedness
in the world when he writes about suture and narrative composure.

Redman (2005) focuses on a small number of related concepts
which he believes are highly relevant to the debate around narrative
and construction of identity. These are *performativity*; *suture*; *persons* and
narrative composure. Narrative composure, originating in Dawson's
(1994) cultural analysis of the adventure genre, is directly related to
the narrative formation of identity. Suture refers to the 'means by which
the "subject" is said to "appear within" or be "stitched into" language'
(Redman, 2005: 31). He provides an examination of a young man who
is in love (Mills and Boon narrative), whom we might view in both
the process of adjustment and liberation. 'Narrating himself from the
positions of both the narrating subject and the subject of narration,
Nick is (however temporarily) able to occupy a moment of *suture* of
seductive depth' (Redman, 2005: 32). 'The position of narrating subject
makes available an apparently stable resting place for identity, a point
of fixity and coherence from which meaning is authored' (Redman, 2005:
32). This concept was used extensively in 1988 by Cohan and Shires
in their investigation into how the person comes to inhabit the identity positions made available within narrative texts.

The notion of a mask or a false self-system is something that has been
explored across psychological, social, anthropological and biological
literature. One of the main questions is why we would need to create
a false self in order to be in the world and why this should matter to
narrative researchers. In fact it is quite relevant to narrative research
in that just as patients can either be compliant or unpopular (see, for
example, Stockwell, 1972), so too can research participants.

The patient comes to healthcare often with a narrative that is dis-
connected and incomplete, disrupted, which is worked on in the
narrative encounter until a more satisfying account emerges along with
the organismic self and the true self.

Narrative and identity are also linked through language. Klein points
out the significance of language in the narrating process, saying that
'Consciousness plays an important role in differentiating and integrating
regions of the self. Or rather, our ability to use language is important'
(1987: 185). She goes on to add that 'we talk to ourselves in words, we
can give an account to ourselves of our world, of our place in it – we
are conscious, we are conscious of ourselves. We can construct verbal
versions of our experiences'.

A verbal version of ourselves may leave some things out which we actually experience and may include things which were not experienced, for example, particular needs and emotions. The use of language and words is vital to the integration of our self-experience; it is also relevant to the use of space within the therapeutic partnership. Archakis and Tzanne (2005) in their narrative study of young people demonstrate how linguistic and conversational choices can be seen as acts of identity in which individuals not only position themselves, but also position themselves in relation to other subcultures, which can either be legitimated or de-legitimated through the narrative.

Power, authority and identity

Power and authority are linked not only to the development of the personal self through relationship: a sense of 'having a voice' is also bound up in cultural (hi)stories. Some cultures, for example, have grown up with subordination and systematic oppression as the norm, leading them to internalise a sense of personal and cultural impotence. Okri (1997), in his work *A Way of Being Free*, addresses the issue of cultural narration with eloquence and passion, focusing on the loss of imagination and creativity which is often a product of such oppression. This loss can be experienced as death itself. Freshwater claims that 'there are many ways to die and not all of them have to do with the extinction of life. Many of them have to do with living . . . the life imposed on you' (2000: 483). One could question from where the process of imposition is initiated: intrapsychically, interpersonally, culturally, or, most likely, all three.

Gender, culture and collective identity

When referring to the self and identity, developed in and through relationship and social context, we are speaking not only of personal identity but also of collective identity that is formed over time within cultures and across societies. Cultural identity is of course important and validated through narrative and storytelling practices. Barton (2004: 519), for example, writes about the role of narrative inquiry in developing culturally competent scholarship. Defining it as an adaptable methodology for valuing co-participation and appreciation of cultural context, she observes: 'Based on the sharing of perspectives, narrative inquiry allows for the experimentation into creating new forms of knowledge'. Barton (2004: 525), in her narrative research with indigenous populations, claims that 'As a methodology congruent with Aboriginal epistemology, narrative inquiry could be about witnessing an insurgent effort by Aboriginal people to reclaim confidence in their identities, regain a political voice, and heal from colonial injustices of the past. It is about a whole life.'

Just as culture is a significant concept in regard to the self, so is gender. Further, both concepts have specific meanings in the context of narrative research. Overcash (2004: 16) suggests that organising concepts around a central topic is a more feminine way of narrating a story. In contrast, more masculine tellings generally follow a more linear succession of events. However, as Overcash explains, this should not be taken literally: communication styles are not sex specific.

Society is a powerful teacher in the construction of the social self. Both social self and society determine which emotions are 'reasonable' to express and which ones are not. One might argue that narrative is a socially and politically engaged tool, teaching society something about the way in which personhood is constructed and how relationships are formed. Indeed, one could ask what and how is narrative contributing to the construction of the social self and society itself?

Transformation of self through narrative and emotion

Narrative researchers have an awareness of the potentially transformatory elements of their research interaction, understanding that 'every interaction is a possible intervention' (Freshwater, 2003). Here we begin to get a sense of some of the skills required of the researcher to foster the appropriate alliances for narrative research to reach its (unlimited) potential. These skills will be addressed more fully in Chapter 13 where we will discuss the importance of research alliance that is grounded in the facilitation and expression of feelings. However, it is important to mention the significance of emotions in narrative research. Both McLeod (1997) and Priest (2000) view storytelling and narrative as an emotionally powerful experience.

Emotions mature through the normal process of socialisation, in which the bonds of intimacy previously limited to mother are extended to an increasingly wider group. This is similar to the interactive pattern between mother and infant, in which new patterns of social discourse are learnt primarily through communication. Attunement now includes social play, control and following implicit rules, which are all communicated through language. The sense of attunement is also used to read other people's direct and indirect non-verbal language, what Casement (1985) terms the unconscious communication in which the participant signifies to the researcher the emotional tone of the relationship.

Clarkson suggests that awareness is a form of experiencing. 'It is the process of being in a vigilant contact with the most important event in the individual/environment.' She goes on to say that 'it is a meaning making function which helps to unify disparate pieces of self-knowledge or consciousness' (1989: 32). It is a route to healing splits and gaps, paving the path towards integration (Klein, 1987).

For the individual who struggles to make contact with the environment and is subsequently not fully aware of their needs and emotions, life can appear bland, with the environment lacking in specific detail, sometimes motivating the move towards an adjustment or liberation narrative of the self. In this case, then, the awareness of emotional needs acts as a spur to transformation, driving individuals towards a willingness to be open in order that they might meet their emergent need and revitalise their own personal narrative.

Summary

Humans have a strong propensity to think of events in a narrative form, whether this is through cultural habit or psychological impulse. We have outlined some of the issues concerning the existence of a narrating self and the relationship of this to the subject of the narrative. Narrative is linked not simply to individual identity but also to communities, cultures and nations. Gender, power and authority also affect the stories people tell.

Collecting, Analysing and Presenting Data

5 Ethical and Political Implications of Narrative Research

Much of the debate around social science research relates to the relationship between the researcher and the researched. Although there is a tendency to focus on doing no harm to participants, the long term consequences are not always easy to calculate. Sumner (2006) writes of the rights to privacy, informed consent and confidentiality in research as being some of the most difficult assurances to give to any participant.

Ethical dilemmas are endemic in all research; however, interactive and relational research such as narrative intensifies the concerns. Of course numerous guidelines have been published and are available freely to any researcher undertaking fieldwork. However, guidelines are just that: they are not obligatory and are difficult to police, bearing in mind that they are open to individual interpretation and application. Ethical values themselves are not absolutes, and one can understand the problems of translating abstract and disputable principles into a set of practical and relevant guidelines to suit a variety of researchers and research settings.

It could be argued that it is impossible to undertake research without some ethical infringement; however, the researcher must, in conjunction with peers and colleagues, make some moral judgements about the balance between the benefits of the research (the need to make known) and the rights of others. (This goes back to Chapter 4.) Sumner (2006: 98) suggests one should 'balance the need to obtain valid data against the rights of the individuals and groups to privacy and autonomy'.

Having already acknowledged that research with human beings is led by guidelines and codes, and that the application of those codes is also contextual, we shall now turn our attention to the ethical and political implications of narrative research, about which very little has been written. This is particularly interesting given that narrative research is itself deemed to be a political and activist activity that quite often explicates complex ethical and moral dilemmas.

Braud and Anderson (1998), in their essay on ethical and political responsibility, propose that making progress for the good of all people requires at least three essential characteristics:

- Recognition of our actions that harm others and an expression of appropriate remorse
- An amendment of harmful actions and their consequences
- Change in future actions

We relate these to our earlier points about knowing self (see Chapters 4 and 13) and the significance of the ability to reflect on one's own practice. Rather than simply presenting guidelines for the ethical use of research skills, Braud and Anderson (1998) also refer to the need to respect the limits of the research. They describe situations when the research is culturally deemed inappropriate, when the research is personally deemed inappropriate, and when the researcher is confronting the ineffable.

Elliott (2005), in her chapter on ethics in narrative research, divides the discussion for the sake of clarity, dealing first with ethics and secondly with political issues. The ethical dimension is defined as issues relating to the relationship between the researcher and participant and the impact of the research process on individuals directly involved in the research. The political dimension is defined as being the broader implications of research, namely the impact on society or subgroups in society.

In more detail Elliott (2005) suggests that the researcher enters into a personal and moral relationship with the participant during data collection, analysis and dissemination. She focuses her attention on the full research process: data collection, informed consent, the potential impact of the research encounter on the participant and additionally on the implications of using narrative with regard to confidentiality and anonymity during analysis and dissemination. The latter can be quite complex, especially given the propensity for direct knowing of information about events and people not immediately connected to the researcher but nevertheless known.

Narrative interviewing brings with it a range of interesting but challenging issues for consideration. Moves away from structured interview techniques over the last two decades and to providing participants with the opportunity to relate narratives about aspects of their lives and experiences as a means of empowering the participant, whilst commendable, do raise questions regarding the nature of the research relationship, specifically the blurring of boundaries between the expert (i.e. researcher) and the storyteller.

Issues regarding the exploitation of the research relationship (specifically related to the power dynamic) have been the topic of debate for many years. Narrative research does have the potential to provide the opportunity for the participant to have a form of control over the data that are collected. Rather than the researcher asking the questions they want to ask, the participants are both the 'subjects and objects in the construction of sociological knowledge' (Graham, 1984: 118). Ochberg (1996: 97) argued that questionnaires provide a narrow menu of selected foci, but that narrative lets participants choose the events that matter to them. Although this is theoretically true, there is still a potential for exploitation, and as with all research, the assumption of equality and reciprocity cannot be taken for granted or assumed.

Finch (1984) discusses the ethics of interviewing groups of women in their own homes in an informal manner in which the research took on an informal, intimate character. Although this form of data collection is effective, it can leave the participant open to exploitation as narrators often disclose confidential and intimate information and the researcher can only provide fairly flimsy guarantees of confidentiality. In addition, when working with participants in their own homes, it is inevitable that the researcher learns much more than what is said in words.

Any research experience could prove positive or negative for the participant. In narrative research there is the possibility that, through sharing a narrative on an unpleasant situation (and/or an unresolved situation), raw emotions may arise; however, an informal, intimate conversation could also provide a safe and positive opportunity for the participants to describe their experience to someone who is interested and listening to their experience. From the latter viewpoint, narrative encounters can be healing and provide a therapeutic environment within which a transformation can begin or be supported (see Chapters 2 and 13).

In their research Proctor and Padfield (1999) found that interviewees had little recall about the interview when subsequently re-interviewed, but interestingly remembered it being a positive experience. There are few empirical accounts of how interviewees perceive and experience interviews. It is acknowledged that the presentation of 'self' within the interview is partly a function of the interview interaction itself, but there is little evidence related to the extent and effect of the interview. As we have previously discussed, the construction of the self (as both interviewee and interviewer) is closely linked to narrative constructions of identity, narrative composure and performativity (see Chapter 4).

Ethics, narrative identity and informed consent

The fact that autobiographical or ontological narratives not only describe a world but also are inseparable from the self raises additional ethical issues. Smythe and Murray (2000: 317) emphasise the traditional conception of research as tapping into a source of data. However, this research model gives rise to ethical principles related to obtaining informed consent from people who are 'giving away' their data to the researcher, and the researcher in turn dealing with the data respectfully.

Narrative is not only descriptive but constitutes the self, thus the research has the potential to be a significant transformational experience. This must be recognised. Narrative ethics are quite different from statistical ethics; personal narratives deal with an individual's meaning of life experiences and personal identity. The information cannot be dissociated from fundamental human values and meaningful life experiences (Smythe and Murray, 2000: 318).

Narrative research has components of research and therapy; as such, ethics from within both fields need to apply (Lieblich, 1996: 173). Personal narratives are bound up with personal identities, raising important questions regarding the analysis of the narrative and in turn the impact of the analysis on the participant.

Mishler (1986a: 119) argues that people can be moved, through their narrative, to the possibility of action. This approach links with the concept of therapy in which (re)formation of the client's self-narratives can occur. There are references to the therapeutic nature of narrative biographical interviews and the possibility of less positive outcomes. Day-Sclater (1998) suggests that the 'effects of interviewing on the self-concept of interviewer and interviewee must be considered'.

Ethics and narrative analysis

It is not only the interview process that can have an effect on the participant but also the way in which the data are interpreted and analysed (positively or negatively). If personal narratives are seen as a central process by which people comprehend and give meaning to their lives and establish a unified coherent sense of self, the deconstruction and interpretation of the narratives (if not done sensitively) may undermine the work being done by the participants to maintain an ontological security (Borland, 1991). Smythe and Murray (2000: 321) state that once the researcher's account of the data is taken as the authoritative interpretation, the participants' understanding of their experience is compromised. Narrative research can become intrusive and damaging, even when participants respond positively.

Confidentiality

Although confidentiality is a basic premise in all research and indeed in healthcare *per se*, within the realm of narrative research it raises unique issues. Because of the holistic and contextual nature of such research, it becomes very difficult for the researcher to ensure anonymity. This is also an issue for longitudinal studies as the data often need to be conceptualised using a case history which may make it possible for the participants to be identified by those who know them. To a degree this problem is resolved by obtaining informed consent and providing clear information to the participant. Whilst some participants do not mind being identified, others clearly do. A further aspect arises when there are unexpected responses should a participant be identified after the research has been published.

On the other hand, some individuals may feel that confidentiality and anonymity deprive them of the chance to have their voices heard within the research. Narrative research therefore contains many more ethical considerations than structured surveys. In a structured survey interview there is a clear contract between researcher and participant. The boundaries of narrative are far less clear than those of the structured survey, but this should not put off the would-be narrative researcher or detract from the use of narrative, rather it should serve as a precursor to high quality, ethically sensitive, meaningful research.

Narrative and the politics of research

Narrative research can be viewed as an appropriate method to give a voice to marginalised groups within society. Empowering participants to engage in narrative can be a liberating experience for individuals and groups. Indeed, many social scientists consider narrative approaches to be popular because of their potential to be subversive or transformative. From a feminist perspective contextual data containing accounts of experience can provide the most useful evidence of the oppressive structures that maintain the power differentials within a society (Smith, 1987; Harding, 1992; Hartsock, 1997).

In contrast Mott and Condor (1997: 64) argue that individuals are not always able to see and understand general systems of inequality from the perspective of their everyday lives. The authors maintain that social facts often exist at a level of statistical abstraction to which the individual has no direct access. Gender discrimination, for example, might become apparent when aggregate data are available, but may not be evident when individual cases are examined. They argue that individual narratives are 'not always subversive or transformative of existing power differentials in society'. People might not be conscious of the aspects of life histories they share with others, and although narratives are important, they do not provide a simple panacea.

Narratives provide an insight into individual lives but provide no guarantee of resolving inequalities; in fact they may even contribute to, rather than undermine, societal inequalities. Atkinson (1997: 212) notes: 'we are as likely to be shackled by the stories we tell (or that are culturally available for our telling) as we are by the form of oppression they might seek to reveal.' The stories people tell can reinforce the make-up of the social fabric which shapes individuals' lives and behaviour. Individual narrative will, therefore, not always be emancipatory.

All discourse will to some extent maintain and reflect the dominant threads of the social fabric, and therefore all research (including non-narrative methods) is in danger of supporting and reproducing the existing power differentials.

Specific features of narratives that allow the maintenance of the hegemony and status quo include:

- The sequential/chronological nature of narrative and the assumption that narrative contains implicit assumptions regarding causal links. As the causal links are not explicit, they are difficult to challenge/debate.
- Narratives use general understandings of the social world, while depicting specific individuals in specific contexts. They reproduce without making specific connections between events and cultural assumptions or social structures. Many assumptions underlying a narrative remain unacknowledged and unchallenged.
- Narratives present a version of the world in terms of the individual's own motivation and local conditions.
- Ewick and Silbey (1995: 219) make distinction between 'hegemonic tales' and 'subversive stories'. Hegemonic tales are narratives that obscure linkages between particular individual experiences and broader social structures. Subversive stories recount particular experiences as rooted in and part of an encompassing cultural, material and political world that extends beyond the local.

Although subversive stories provide a critique of the social world, it is possible for the researcher to use hegemonic tales as a collective narrative to reveal what is taken for granted in a society. The researcher has the responsibility of providing an analysis of narratives which makes explicit that which has gone without saying, and makes links between particular cases and underlying social conditions.

By revealing what is being taken for granted within a society, narrative research can provide a subversive story about people's lives and experiences, placing the narratives within the social and cultural context and making explicit the specific resources which have been used to structure them.

Smythe and Murray (2000: 327) refer to 'typal narratives'. These are the narratives that social scientists construct and relate broader psychological and social themes. They provide concrete examples of theoretical constructs developed by social scientists. The difference between typal and personal narratives highlights why some participants may feel that the research does not do them justice as complex and unique individuals.

Participants do not expect that their personal views would be apparent in a quantitative study, but perhaps because of the informal, intimate situation in which the narrative is produced, the interpersonal relationship between researcher and participant, and the generally small sample, individuals feel that their life and experience should be represented holistically. This expectation may also be a result of the relationship between researcher and participant, in which they are led to believe that their narrative will be presented as part of the research and the integrity of their accounts will be preserved.

Participants may well be disconcerted that the researcher does not appear interested in the content but in the cultural discourses or narrative strategies. Appreciation of narrative is an art form and narrative needs to answer critical and analytical questions; the researcher needs to meet the challenge of collecting the narrative material without exploiting the individuals who have consented to provide detailed biographical accounts of their lives/experiences.

Narrative as constructing ethics

Abma (1999: 171) suggests that people tell each other stories to find out how they should act in certain situations, how they relate to others, and what their identity and role are. We referred to the creation of identity in Chapter 4; here we relate this to the development of the ethical self. 'In telling stories, actors are involved in the act of generating *value*, judging the worth of people's lives and social practices' (Abma, 1999: 171). Narratives often embed examples of actions and the consequences of those actions. This is relevant not only to clinical and professional practice but also of course to the impact of our behaviours on others and on society. As such, narratives contain a moral framework (link to ethics). Standard stories are created, one of which is that the self can and should act ethically, and not least the self of the researcher.

Summary

All research raises certain ethical, moral and political questions for the researcher. Guidelines for undertaking ethical research exist across a variety of professional disciplines. Just as each research method has its own unique features, so does narrative research, not least in regard to ethics. The sensitive and often intimate nature of the researcher–participant relationship, along with the personal and often complex data collected, require that the researcher pay specific attention to ways in which the relationship and findings could be exploited.

6 The Proposal for a Narrative Study

The proposal for a narrative research project differs slightly, though not much, from other types of protocol. The researcher needs to explain the research in some detail and justify it, as many funding bodies and even academics may not know the narrative approach as well as other types of qualitative inquiry; the specific advantages of narrative research need to be pointed out to the readers. Apart from explaining these details, the proposal writer can take the traditional route of 'selling' the proposed research. For acceptance of the proposal the researcher needs to justify the research and show that it is both important and urgent. A short glossary or an explanation of terms is also useful for the readers of the proposal, and it can be placed somewhere in the beginning or in an appendix.

Punch (2000: 22) focuses on the main elements of the research proposal and suggests several questions to which we will add:

- What is the topic of the proposed research? (What is the research question?)
- What does the researcher want to find out and learn from the research? (What will the researcher know at the end of the research?)
- How will he or she get to fulfil the aim of the research? (What are the process and the method?)

Why this question, why this topic, why narrative inquiry?

There is one major difference between the proposal in quantitative and qualitative inquiry: Sandelowski and Barosso (2003) argue that proposal writing in qualitative research presents a challenge to any researcher as the research develops over time. The narrative research proposal too is generally tentative and not determined for all time. The researchers cannot specify exactly how the inquiry will proceed because the stories are, to a large extent at least, in the control of the participants, and the research must not be formulaic. Most grant-holding bodies and indeed ethics committees demand that researchers make firm statements and describe the process with clarity. In narrative inquiry, however, it must be made explicit that the research will be evolving throughout the process and that the questions and content specified in the proposal might change and develop. Many funding bodies, agencies and ethics committees are not comfortable with this, so the researcher has to explain that the research questions are not tightly fixed for all time but may emerge, and become more focused and specific in the process of the research.

Readers of the protocol have to appraise whether the proposer is capable of doing the research and is knowledgeable about the methods, whether it is viable within the boundaries of topic, time and location and whether it is worthwhile – and useful. The latter is difficult to judge as the inquiry might have no direct outcomes and its value can only emerge over time or on the completion of similar studies in the field.

The research question or problem

To write a proposal, the researcher needs a *research question* (or questions) that is significant in healthcare inquiry and that has not been asked before in the same way or within the same sampling frame, or in the same circumstances or setting. For instance, the topic of 'living with diabetes' might have been explored often, but the issue of young adolescents or old people who live with diabetes could be examined in a different way or in a different geographical and cultural environment. If a large amount of knowledge already exists about the proposed area of study, narrative research is not appropriate.

Researchers are not always clear whether they wish to answer a research question or solve a research problem. Punch (2000) explains the difference. A research question emerges when a researcher asks the question: What do I want to find out; what question do I want to answer? A research problem is a puzzle that emerges directly from a concern in the clinical or educational setting in need of solution, sometimes concerned with outcomes. Of course there is overlap between the two, but in narrative inquiry the researcher usually deals with research questions initially although the answer may solve problems.

Usually the research problem or question in the healthcare field emerges naturally from the clinical or educational world of the health professional or academic, but sometimes researchers might have to search for a suitable topic which arises from a puzzle or urgent issue in healthcare. For instance, a nursing lecturer might wish to examine a problem in education and finds that the area of action learning is of special interest and has topicality; hence he or she will focus on this topic.

The research question or problem generally determines methods; hence narrative researchers seek to find the answers to specific questions. As in other types of qualitative study there is no hypothesis, though, of course, assumptions exist. The researchers have to uncover their pre-suppositions and experiences in the area of the proposed project but hold them at bay at the same time so as not to prejudice the study. Creswell (2003) suggests that researchers generally pose one 'central' or key question and a number of sub-questions rather than stating objectives. In narrative inquiry the key question focuses directly on the main phenomenon to be explored. No narrative research is successful if the question is not interesting for the researcher or significant for the profession. It is essential that the proposal indicate that the problem has been clearly understood and that the research, when completed, will at least point towards a solution to the problem or an answer to the question. Examples of research questions are as follows:

- What do people experience when they are diagnosed with . . . (a specific condition)?
- How do people cope with chronic illness?
- The transition from well person to a patient with arthritis
- Becoming and being a person with diabetes
- Living and coping with bowel cancer
- How do people with mental illness experience physical healthcare?

The researcher states *the aim* of the study after having decided on a research question and recognised the gaps that exist in the field of study. To persuade others of the significance of their aim, researchers have to state it clearly. All too often, novice researchers are so enthusiastic about their proposed narrative study that they do not state a clear aim. Defining the aim means stating what will be found out and achieved by the research itself, and may or may not be linked to the eventual purpose of this research. For instance: 'to improve diabetes care' is not a research aim but a potential outcome. The aim of this type of research might be: 'to explore the experience of people with diabetes (in order to improve diabetes care)'. Another example of an aim might be the development of an evidence based assessment tool for identification and assessment of self-harming behaviours in young men. The research part is to study the evidence and then use it to develop the tool. Detailed objectives have no place in narrative inquiry as they would tie down the researcher and structure the study too rigidly from the beginning rather than keeping its developmental character.

The *title* of the proposed research needs to be carefully chosen. It has to capture the interest of the reader, and reflect its aim and content without being a clever journalistic catch phrase which research committees or funding bodies might not take seriously. An overly long title will not attract readers. Terms such as 'aspects of', 'a study of', etc., are redundant as it is obvious that this is a study or aspects of particular phenomena – though many researchers feel comfortable with the phrase 'a study of'. Students writing a dissertation or thesis may come back to the title at a later stage as the full content of the study is not determined beforehand owing to the nature of narrative research and it can change in the process. They have to take care, however, to read the guidelines of the university. Our own university, for instance, does not allow change in title once the 'intention to submit' has been sent to the examinations office. Examples of some titles (not all from actual studies) are as follows:

- The emotional experience of undergoing an operation
- Patient narratives from an orthopaedic ward
- Mothers, fathers and gender: parental narratives about children (Peterson, 2004)
- Identity commitments in personal stories of mental illness on the internet (Jones R.A., 2005)
- Silence in court: the devaluation of the stories of nurses in the narratives of health law (Chiarella, 2000)
- Premature death by suicide in the adolescent rural population

The titles for external funding bodies are generally straightforward and simple, and show that the researcher is focused on a specific issue, for instance: 'The elderly person's experience of acute hospital care.'

The rationale of the project and the initial literature review

In the introduction to the study, the researcher justifies the research by explaining *why* it is necessary, important and urgently needed. This is the *rationale* of the study. Here the context, setting and background have to be explained. The major concepts being used also need exploring (see Chapter 9). Hart (1998: 188) advises describing the type of problem and its extent by giving examples. He also suggests that the proposal writer show the relevance of the research for the profession and patients, and for the health service, as well as pointing to the potential consequences if it is not carried out.

The *initial literature review* is a summary of the research work that has been carried out in the past in this particular topic area. In narrative inquiry the literature review should not be too detailed as it might force the researchers into a particular direction instead of listening to the stories and taking their clues from the participants. Wolcott (2001) and Glaser (1978, 1999) claim that a long exhaustive literature review in qualitative research is not necessary; indeed it would be too directive. Glaser suggests broad background reading but warns researchers to avoid the literature that is closely linked to their specific studies and which should only be perused when it becomes relevant during the research process. This would also be advisable for narrative inquiry.

We would argue, however, that in the proposal the current state of knowledge must be explored to demonstrate where gaps occur that the researcher wishes to fill, and that the proposed project does not duplicate the work of others. The study needs to be located among other, similar studies, and the researcher has to show how it will differ from them, as well as to describe what issues other writers have discussed as a result of their own research. Indeed the initial review is necessary to clarify the aim of the research and critically evaluate the research of others in relation to the proposed research. The in-depth literature review, however, is not part of the proposal and will be left for a later stage. Researchers do need to demonstrate to the readers of the proposal that they are knowledgeable about qualitative research by explaining why the literature review is not exhaustive. It is also important to make this explicit to those who do not know about narrative research – and there may be persons on the panel who judge the proposal who lack this expertise.

The significance of the proposed research to nursing

The question is whether what was learnt from the research is something new or different that is really worth knowing, and could be useful for the clinical setting. 'Blue skies' research, the type of inquiry which does not result in direct practical applications and practical knowledge, rarely finds favour with grant or funding bodies, and, although it is possible for academic purposes, nursing research has a greater chance of being accepted if its potential outcomes have clear implications for professional practice or education.

The nurse researcher has to justify the study and the effort and money spent on it by explaining what importance it has for patients/ the health service/professionals/education, etc. The *outcomes* of the research, which many agencies expect to be stated, can, of course, not be clearly determined from the outset of narrative research, but its potential *use and implications* should be made explicit.

It is noteworthy that Locke et al. (2000) distinguish between research that is carried out to 'understand' something and that which is done to 'improve' something. In most nursing research, however, both goals are important, although finding out and understanding are the first step in the process and the stated aim reflects this. For instance, a practice nurse might carry out research on parents' decision-making processes concerning having their children immunised by the controversial MMR (measles, mumps and rubella) vaccine. This research would be carried out to better understand the parents' reasons for not immunising their children, in order to enhance communication with healthcare professionals.

Practical considerations

Researchers need to show that the project is possible within the time-frame and that it is feasible within the resources that are at their disposal. The *timeline* is usually divided into segments of tasks, but the sections often overlap; in these types of research projects data collection and analysis sometimes overlap and the literature review is overarching and ongoing throughout the research. It is, of course, desirable that researchers demonstrate their credibility as professionals and their knowledge as qualitative, narrative researchers. This can be shown in appropriate statements and through the references at the end of the proposal.

Design, procedures and process

There will be enough information about the methodology, design and procedures to show that they are appropriate and valid. Researchers always have a plan for their research and show how this plan is put into practice: what strategies will be adopted to achieve the completion of the plan. The procedures include sampling as well as data collection and analysis. The very first step is to place the research within the qualitative 'paradigm', a term – often overused – in research, meaning a world view or 'a set of assumptions about the world' (Punch, 2000: 35). The extent of this debate depends on the readers of the research (usually an academic proposal for a PhD thesis needs to be more extensive and explicit on this than a proposal for a grant-giving body). The question that has to be answered is why this study is specifically based on the participants' narratives and not on other sources of data. It is important for the researcher to clarify and make explicit that the research is inductive in character; that is, it proceeds from specific instances to general statements rather than the reverse. The data collected by the researcher have priority.

Researchers discuss whom they include and exclude in the *sample* and for what reasons they do so. In narrative research the sample need not be large as it is based on information-rich cases, and indeed the inclusion criteria might be fairly narrow. Researchers always explain how they gain access to the sample. The strategy of gaining access to the sample has to be described, something that novice researchers often forget. As agencies in the health service and ethics committees deal most often with quantitative research, researchers need to justify small samples.

The readers of the proposal would expect the researcher to tell them about the *delimitations* and *limitations* of the research. Delimitations are the boundaries of the population investigated within which the research takes place. Limitations are its potential weaknesses and constraints, and the researcher has to make explicit the reasons for these.

In narrative research the only *data sources* are people's stories, usually in spoken words, although written stories would also be possible. The *analysis* of data needs to be discussed in a fair amount of detail so that readers can evaluate the methods and procedures used.

Last, the issues of validity or *trustworthiness* are explored by the researcher. He or she must show that the research will be credible and present the reality of the participants and that the findings or theoretical ideas generated by the study will be transferable to other, similar cases. Other researchers will be able to apply the criteria of trustworthiness at the completion of the study. A clear *audit trail* is necessary (see Chapters 9 and 10).

Although the proposal has to demonstrate the ability of the researcher to think clearly, to write with authority and to make decisions on the basis of reading expert papers and making judgements, the final account will probably be quite different from the proposal, because the process and outcomes of narrative research can never be wholly predicted.

Ethical issues

The proposal also needs a short discussion of *ethical considerations*, potential problems in this arena, and how they would be resolved. Researchers must make clear that they have obtained or will apply for ethics committee approval. Most importantly, however, it has to be demonstrated that the researcher has considered ethical issues and will implement an ethical approach (see Chapter 5).

Summary

The narrative proposal for nursing contains the following elements:

- The background and justification of the research including the important research question

- The aim of the study – what it wants to achieve
- An initial short literature review of the field which shows the conceptual framework and points to the gaps in knowledge
- The design and procedures that the researcher intends to use – i.e. what is the plan and the process of the research
- The significance of the research for clinical practice
- The limits and delimitations of the research
- Potential use of the knowledge gained from the study in the nursing arena
- The manner of dissemination of the findings

Although there are similarities with proposals in other types of qualitative research, it is important to point out the uniqueness of narrative inquiry.

7 The Art of Sampling and Collecting Data

Sampling and data collection are closely related. Data can only be gathered once a sample has been chosen. The type of sample influences the depth, breadth and quality of data although these factors do not always determine the quality of the final account.

The sample is usually decided on before data collection takes place, but sampling can also be an ongoing process where a researcher adds participants when new ideas and concepts emerge and can be followed up, like theoretical sampling in grounded theory. However, it must be clear that people are not the only 'sampling units': particular phenomena, time periods, events or incidents can also be the unit of sampling, although in narrative research human beings more commonly constitute the sample. For instance, in a study of the emotional experience of old people in hospital, old people form the main sampling unit. The researcher might, however, also sample critical events, accidents or periods of interaction.

Identifying and selecting potential participants

The participants chosen must be an appropriate sample so that the aim of the research will be achieved. Appropriate people are those who belong to the type of person from whom the researcher wishes to acquire knowledge because they have experience and information about the phenomenon, or who best represent the group which is being studied. This means the selection of a criterion-based or purposive sample: the potential participants should meet the particular criterion or criteria which the researcher selected at the time of developing the research question. For instance, a nurse who wishes to explore the experience of low back pain might select a small sample of individuals who visit the practice of a general practitioner, or who attend a pain clinic for a back pain problem. Of course, individuals differ in the amount and nature of their experience and the researcher can take this into account. There might be a mix of participants with long-term problems or those who have less experience of a condition. The researcher might choose instead from a group of those who have had a specific condition, experience or treatment over a long time. Where particular knowledge and experience of the phenomenon are required, the sample consists of 'information-rich' cases. The researcher needs to demonstrate that these have 'typicality', meaning they represent the particular group that has knowledge and experience of the phenomenon. Though the sample might have typicality, it must be remembered that the researcher does not claim generalisability for the eventual findings but wishes to understand and explore the meanings of a particular group of people. In this respect, sampling in narrative research is similar to that in other forms of qualitative inquiry. However, there is a problem in narrative research: participants need to be able to articulate their feelings and thoughts. In interviews that are interactive, researchers can help participants to articulate, but, when listening to long stories, holding the thread and simultaneously facilitating participants' attempts to express their thoughts might be more difficult. Inarticulate individuals who are not able to tell stories coherently might not be included in the sample. Clearly this is an issue when working with disabled people or with those whose first language is not English. Their stories, however, are just as important, or even more so, as those of people who can talk easily and fluently. The quality of data also depends on the researcher's skills in dealing with these stories, filling some of the gaps and, in particular, connecting with the participants.

Sample size

Sampling in narrative research can rely on a very small number of people as depth rather than breadth in data collection is sought, although Mason (2002) suggests that there is no particular reason why it has to be small. The number included depends on the research question, focus and aim of the research, and whether the research question can be answered. It is obvious that a larger sample is needed when various groups of people are involved in the research rather than when the sample is homogeneous. For instance, if researchers wish to obtain stories from patients, nurses and doctors, the sample needs to be larger than when they collect and analyse patient stories only. The quality of information, however, is more important than numbers in the sample. In any case, the researcher does not search for generalisability. As Patton (2002: 245) states about all qualitative research: 'The validity, meaningfulness and insights of qualitative inquiry have more to do with the information richness of the cases selected and the observational/analytical capabilities of the researcher than with sample size.' There is no fixed sample size in narrative research, though novice researchers always attempt to find the optimum number before they start. The size depends on the phenomenon or group under study and the rationale of the research. For example, in an in-depth and longitudinal study of the process of therapeutic change in psychotherapy, a sample of four clients generated sufficient data. In contrast, a narrative analysis of the use of internet chat rooms by straight men and their subsequent risk-taking behaviours had a sample exceeding 40.

The single sampling unit

Of course, the sampling unit in narrative research need only consist of one single individual whom the researcher sees as appropriate as a special case or as an illuminative or illustrative case for the phenomenon under study (though 'case' is not a good choice of word as it tends to objectify the participant). It might be the narrative of an individual who has a rare condition, inhabits a particular place in society or is a carer or professional with expert knowledge. Specific accounts based on the individual's story can then be made. The researcher has to demonstrate that the 'single case' sample is justifiable and give good reasons for it. The choice of one case or very few, makes the selection quite straightforward as long as the researcher can justify the reasons for the small sample in the research.

Todres and Galvin (2005) justify the idea of a single case study. They suggest that this is about focus on unique details and context, and not necessarily breadth. Although the findings of this type of study are not generalisable to a larger population, the ideas of the phenomenon under investigation can be transferable to other cases as it is about 'authenticity' of human experience. The authors (Galvin et al., 2005) illustrate this in their writing about one carer's experience with Alzheimer's. This research is based on an intimate carer's journey and his unique role of carer and advocate for a relative with Alzheimer's.

Types of sampling

Purposive and single case sampling – the latter also being a type of purposeful sampling – are only examples of sampling. Holloway and Wheeler (2002), Patton (2002) and Ritchie et al. (2003) discuss a number of sampling types apart from these. We shall describe the types that are most common in narrative inquiry. Most of these sampling types are variations of purposive sampling.

A *typical case sample* includes 'normal' or 'average' cases or events that happen frequently. For example, one of our colleagues singled out 'typical' individuals from a large survey which had been carried out and used narrative interviews to hear their stories. The findings from this sample might have typicality.

Homogeneous sampling includes individuals or phenomena that are similar to each other and have the same characteristics (for the purpose of the study). For instance, the experience of diabetes of women in an ethnic minority group might be explored; this means that gender and ethnic group membership are important criteria for the research. The sample which consists of women with diabetes in this minority group is homogeneous. A sample can be homogeneous merely in one aspect or characteristic, such as, for instance, length of condition, age, occupation or gender.

A *heterogeneous sample* consists of people or phenomena that vary from each other. The researcher wishes to identify these variations. It is obvious that a heterogeneous sample needs to be larger than a homogeneous one. An example from pain studies might show that women, men and children are involved in storytelling, and the researcher is interested in the variations of these groups. *Extreme case and deviant case sampling* means that unusual people or 'contrary occurrences' are selected which do not fit into 'typical' or 'average' mode. In *critical case sampling*, critical incidents or phenomena are chosen, or those individuals who have knowledge and experience of these. For instance, a nurse might want to explore feelings about accidents at work; she will listen to those who have experienced these more frequently than others.

Many researchers, especially neophytes, use *convenience or opportunistic sampling*. They approach people who are easily accessible and take opportunities to sample where the possibility exists. This is not the best type of sampling as it doesn't require much thought but is used when researchers are unable to recruit participants through formal channels. Anyone who fits the criteria might be included. For example, in a study of outcomes of cancer care in rural communities it was not possible to gain access except where the researcher was able to shadow the specialist nurse (ethical guidelines were, of course, followed).

Chain referral sampling is also common. It is a type of sampling in which early participants suggest further individuals who have special knowledge and experience of the area of research. This sampling strategy is sometimes used in the investigation of sensitive topics as the individuals need not be named or identified by professional groups but can talk informally when another participant passes them on to the researcher. An example of this kind of sampling might consist of young people with sexually transmitted diseases who would not always have identified themselves to the health services, or drug users who are reluctant to admit to their habit in a professional–client setting but are prepared to tell their stories informally to a researcher.

(Of course, great care must be taken in this type of sampling, as both the safety of the researcher and the anonymity of the participants are at risk; legal issues have to be considered too.)

We also mentioned above *theoretical sampling*, first developed by Glaser and Strauss – and much used in all types of qualitative inquiry – which is often carried out in grounded theory or ethnographic research. The concepts and issues of importance that emerge are followed up by the researcher who selects new sampling units to examine these. It cannot be planned before the research begins and is an ongoing process. However, this type of sampling is unusual for narrative research and not wholly appropriate: because theoretical sampling often depends on interview interaction, it might interrupt the flow of stories and become too directive (progressively focused).

A total population sample is also a rarity in narrative research, though members of a very small group in a specific location with similar experiences might exist and all be asked to tell their stories. For instance, a group of specialist cancer nurses in a large teaching hospital with similar experiences might agree to become narrators of stories and would make up the total population of cancer nurses in X Hospital.

Researchers can also sample settings or locations. For instance, they might access a number of participants from different types of hospital or indeed from several hospitals or GP practices in different locations; they may access people in micro- or macro-settings. Indeed, the settings may be similar to each other, or they may differ, depending on the goal of the researcher and the research. For instance, if researchers wish to know about the emotional experience of people in hospital, they might collect stories from different types of hospital. They might listen to stories well after the event or during the process of the experience. The latter could, however, create difficulty as participants are more involved in the immediate situation when they inhabit it. They might also be more vulnerable at this time.

Random sampling is a rarity in narrative research where sampling is always purposive or criterion-based in some way. However, when a researcher is able to choose from a very large group of volunteers, he or she sometimes chooses randomly – for instance every third person from the group. This cannot be called random sampling in narrative research as it is initially based on very specific criteria.

Access and negotiation

Initially researchers gain access to participants through the 'gatekeepers', those who control access to the participants. However, participants might also be volunteering in response to a newspaper advertisement, or another type of recruitment. Ethics do demand that the sample consist of voluntary and willing participants who are not coerced in any way (see Chapter 5).

Inclusion and exclusion criteria

Whoever is included in or excluded from the sample depends on the aim of the research. The sample selected should support the researcher's intention as well as having the knowledge and experience needed for the study. Exclusion is determined not only by the knowledge and experience of the research participant but also by traits such as vulnerability – which might make ethical issues problematic – and demographic factors such as, for instance, age, gender or ethnicity. Vulnerable people are often excluded unless their experience is specifically explored. For instance, a researcher might wish to explore the perspectives of new mothers. Those who have problems in the birth process or with their new babies might appropriately be excluded unless they are specifically the focus of the research.

When narrative researchers evaluate their sampling strategies, they might think of the following questions that can be answered in the research report:

- How did I gain access to the participants?
    By newspaper, GP practice or hospital advertisement
    Through mediation by gatekeepers
    Through other health professionals
    Through voluntary agencies
- Who was approached and recruited?
    Voluntary and willing individuals
    A criterion-based or purposive sample
- Which type of sample was selected?
    Homogeneous, heterogeneous
    Critical or deviant case, convenience sample
- What were the limitations of the sample?
    Careful inclusion and exclusion criteria
- Why did I select this particular sample size?
    Depth of narrative material
    Impossibility of finding more volunteers (this is not a good reason and the research plan should be rethought)

The narrative approach to sampling does not demand that the sample be saturated (as it should be in grounded theory). The stories of the people involved in narrative inquiry are unique but also share many elements of common experience in a specific context.

The relationship between researcher and storytellers

The research relationship between the researcher and the other participants is of major importance for a number of reasons, both ethical and practical. The participants should feel confident in the situation and not in awe of the researcher. Even in narrative inquiry where the participants have a great deal of control, there is no real balance of power; the researcher is still in a position of power and cannot exploit participants' vulnerability. Trust and a relationship have to be developed. Russell and Kelly (2002: 4) state that the researcher and the participant should develop sensitivity towards each other and 'foster an I-and-Thou relationship (Buber, 1970) that allows and promotes the humanity of both researcher and participant'. This type of relationship generates reciprocity.

Reciprocity is also important for research purposes: in collaboration, researcher and participants create narrative meaning. Research relationships are always complex and difficult. Participants find a sympathetic listener and a feeling of contributing to research in the clinical field which they know might help later clients of the health service. We found in our own research that not many participants had ever shared their experiences before, and they were glad that somebody gave them this opportunity, particularly as they have a measure of control and are able to follow their own ideas and explore avenues which they had not visited before. For instance, Howarth (2006) found that patients diagnosed with multiple sclerosis appreciated the time given to them in the research process.

As we have argued before, storytelling might also assist in a healing process. Researchers on the other hand gain many advantages, both personal and professional. The most important gain is the usefulness and implications for the clinical setting, but they might also foster their careers through the research.

Collecting data from interviews and other sources

The main and primary sources of data for narrative nursing inquiry are the oral stories of the participants gained in interaction with the researcher; these consist of the unique and individual accounts of people about their own experience. There are, however, other sources of narrative data, for instance diaries, letters or books, but these are accessed less frequently. Narrative research, although imbued with observations of the researcher, does not consist of analyses of participant observation. It relies wholly on spoken and written and occasionally visual data.

How to collect stories

Narrative researchers cannot just go into the research situation and say 'Tell me a story about . . .'. That would mean that they neglect the participant's initial concerns and the research relationship. We call the data collection method for stories 'narrative interviewing' which is well planned and prepared although it does not use a rigid structure or focus on single issues.

The narrative interview

The narrative interview is the tool through which the researcher gains access to the stories of participants. In its simplest form interviewing is a strategy of collecting data in the form of words from participants who are asked to share their experience or lives. For the researcher in healthcare inquiry this means taking a focus on an illness or professional experience, and it may be carried out with health professionals, patients or other groups, or indeed with the 'significant others' of these groups. As we suggested before, the term 'interview' can be misleading as it presupposes frequent interview interaction between researchers and the people from whom they wish to obtain the data. The narrative interview instead is restricted to a small number of questions from the researcher and centres on the flow of talk from the participants. If the researcher interrupts too often, the thread of the story might be lost.

The stories act as filters, of course, and exclude what the participants do not know or want to remember. It is grounded in their own life world or experiences. The way they see the 'truth' of their experiences is enclosed in the stories. The narrative interview is most productive when the interviewer suppresses his or her own desire to speak and helps participants to produce spontaneous talk. Kvale (1996) describes this type of interview as a journey in which the interviewer and the interview partners travel together, and where the latter tell the researcher of their 'lived world'.

Steps in interviewing

The researcher must set up the interview in a congenial setting and needs to have 'people skills' so that the participants can feel at ease and inclined to talk. Of course, the interviewer does not just seek to put the participants at ease so that he or she can obtain better stories; it is also ethically appropriate to help the participants to relive the past without suffering unnecessary stress. None the less, the setting should encourage talk.

Schütze (1977, cited by Jovchelovitch and Bauer, 2000), a German qualitative researcher, suggested that storytelling has its own distinctive mode, starting with revealing events and incidents from the past and uncovering feelings. Jovchelovitch and Bauer (2000) reiterate that tacit rules, 'those which everybody knows', determine the form of talk. They refer to detailed texture, relevance fixation and closure of 'Gestalt' a whole which is greater than its parts. Detailed information from stories is necessary so that the transition from event to event, and incident to incident, can be grasped. The participants tell those stories which have relevance to them and are important from their own perspectives as well as having important links to the topic or phenomenon under study about which they are asked. Storytellers also strive to present a 'Gestalt', so that the listener can grasp it in its entirety. Jovchelovitch and Bauer (2000) advise interviewers not to pre-structure the talk, so that they have minimum control. Only in this situation can stories flourish. This way the participants will be stimulated and encouraged to tell their stories. Preliminary work on the part of the researchers is necessary so that they know something of the phenomenon they wish to research and in doing so grasp participants' stories more easily and quickly. Careful sampling will ensure that the participants have experience and information about the phenomenon in order to develop their stories.

Ways of collecting stories

Czarniawska (2004: 42–44) differentiates the ways in which stories can be collected into three types:

(1)   Recording of spontaneous storytelling
(2)   Eliciting stories
(3)   Asking for stories

First, stories that are being told by chance and informally, during fieldwork and prolonged engagement, are good sources of unexpected data. The second type of story is that told about critical incidents which the researchers themselves 'elicit'. For instance, stories about ward accidents or professional conflict might be obtained from nurses (we are not advocating this for novice researchers as there are numerous ethical problems involved in such research, but include it as an example). The choice of the incident depends on the researcher, of course, but the stories are wholly those of the participants.

The third type of story is asked for specifically by the researcher attempting to access the thoughts and feelings of the participants. This is the most common form as researchers have an agenda, however much they wish to hear about the participants' experiences.

There are some simple ground rules for the collection of narrative data:

- The researcher's agenda should be of importance to the field of nursing and health care.
- The research question should be broad enough so that rich data can be gathered, and focused enough to be examined in depth.
- The area of research should be interesting and significant for the participants so that they are able to explore and narrate their experiences, feelings and thoughts.
- The interviewer should not direct the participants towards specific issues within the area of study but let them emerge naturally through the participants' stories.

Diaries and other sources of data

Diaries or journals are sometimes complements to oral tales. There are two types of participant diary. One is the diary created specifically for the research: the researcher asks participants to record their ongoing experiences in writing. It is kept during the process of the experience that is to be studied. Riley and Hawe (2005), for instance, report on a narrative study which relied on diaries of professionals. Two years of diaries were written by community development officers who worked with recent mothers in primary care to reduce postnatal depression and improve new mothers' physical wellbeing. They were used as a complement to oral stories.

Another type of study uses diaries that are in existence before the research starts and that could be analysed during the research process. Of course, books and letters might also contain participant stories and might be accessed by the researcher long after they were written.

We do not subscribe to Elliott's claim (2005) that narrative research can rely on both qualitative and quantitative elements, though there might be elements of narrative in the latter. Sampling should be purposive and criterion-based, and data collection relatively unstructured to elicit storytelling. Quantitative methods do not seem appropriate for stories told by people. Narrative inquiry is rooted in literary traditions as Elliott herself suggests.

Summary

The chapter includes a discussion of purposive sample. We explained that the sample size need not be large, because it is depth, not breadth, that is sought. Participants need to meet the inclusion and exclusion criteria set by the researcher. A number of sampling types were described.

There are a variety of ways in which data are collected in narrative research, such as narrative interviews and diaries. These data should be rich and explore the area of study in depth. Central to the data collection phase is the relationship between the researcher and the storyteller. The data collection phase and narrative analysis are inextricably linked, although for the purposes of this book and for clarity we have drawn distinctions.

8 Narrative Analysis and Contextualisation

Riessman (2006: 186) defines narrative analysis as 'a family of approaches to diverse kinds of text, which have in common a storied form'. She goes on to point out that what makes these diverse texts narrative is sequence and consequence in which 'events are selected, organised, connected and evaluated as meaningful for a particular audience'. As we have already indicated, there are numerous definitions and conceptualisations of narrative and narrative research. Consequently this leads to different views and indeed methods of analysis. Thus, although all narratives require some sort of interpretation, the manner in which this is undertaken may differ. In this chapter we outline some of the ways in which narrative can be analysed. Drawing upon a variety of philosophical perspectives, we aim to provide practical guidance to the researcher who is interested and intends to conduct narrative analysis. Rather like Riessman (2006), we wish to avoid presenting a hierarchy of approaches to narrative analysis. Moreover we would like to emphasise that the following approaches are not mutually exclusive and can be combined to form a creative and individual analysis pertinent to the data being interpreted.

Narrative data can include both oral and written accounts, both of which are offered in the language, experience and judgement of the storyteller. Narrative researchers take an *empathic* stance towards the data and, as such, researchers and participants can employ both a subjective and an objective overview when engaging with the data. In other words, rather like the concept of empathy, the researcher is involved with the data and the participant, but also keeps one foot on the outside of the interview in order to be able to observe themselves and the participant (and the dialogic process) from a reflexive standpoint (see also Chapter 13). In this sense, the narrative approach attempts to overcome the distance between the knower and the known. When working with data, narrative researchers are not looking for one single and simple truth, rather they are aware that multiple truths co-exist; thus there is no one correct reading or interpretation of the text. Josselson and Lieblich (2001: 280) capture this understanding when they write: 'the narrative research approach is oriented toward subjectivity, intentionality, pluralism, relativism, holism and contextuality'. Using individual narrative to understand collective and shared meanings might be a focus of the analysis. As Frank (2002) asks, from the perspective of conventional science, how can the narrator be considered an ideal type of some larger group or class of people? However, narrative analysis, according to Mishler (1995), renders itself appropriate for theory generation.

Regardless of the actual methods used, the process of collecting data is an active one and one that engages the researcher at different levels. Indeed Moustakas (1990), Braud and Anderson (1998) and Freshwater (1998) comment on how the research question and the data becomes part of the researcher's life in both waking and sleeping moments. These researchers view a period of incubation as critical to the process of analysis and interpretation, suggesting that this invites the creative process to do its work whilst the researcher is in a relaxed and restful state of being and doing *nothing*. Braud and Anderson (1998: 91) say that 'To proceed directly to data analysis without an incubating downtime for the new information to settle and shift in the awareness of the researcher undermines the intuitive process.' They go on: 'The researcher may even wish to return to periods of incubation throughout the data analysis as well, especially if the analysis is lengthy or if the researcher feels stymied at any point.'

When analysing narrative data the analysis should accommodate the data as it presents itself, rather than being determined from the outset. In this sense, data can truly reveal and shape itself (and the participants), whilst the researcher is open to illuminating insights and breakthroughs. 'Narrative analysis requires that we focus on the narrative plot, exploring the potential and limits of each patient's narrative and the process of its construction and the social discourse that helps to maintain it' (Goncalves et al., 2004: 104).

The purpose of the data analysis is to explain how 'meanings, their linkages and horizons, are actively constructed within the interview environment. It is about "deconstructing" the participants' talk. Showing the reader the "hows" or the "whats" of the narrative frames of lived experience' (Holstein and Gubrium, 1995: 79–80), Priest (2000) observes that narrative analysis does not have a single heritage, drawing instead on a diverse range of sources. Limitations with traditional interviews include issues related to form, structure and content, all of which have been used to legitimise the use of unstructured narrative data collection and analysis (Priest, 2000). Making a case for the use of narrative method, Lucas (1997) stresses the retention of context and large pieces of material which should be considered as the units of analysis. Similarly, Josselson and Lieblich (1995: 31) note that narrative analysis provides an alternative to the 'traditional "scientific" understanding of the individual as "abstracted" out of his or her context rather than as part of it' (this is discussed further in regard to holistic and categorical analysis).

Stories are never just representations of experience, they are also interpretations. The process of interpretation imposes an order on the experiences, making analysis and interpretation of narrative text different from the interpretation of scientific text; although we referred to the relationship between causality and narrative in Chapters 1 and 2, in narrative, events are temporally and spatially connected, unlike scientific texts, which are often connected using causal laws.

Thus it is the '*sequentiality* (temporal order of events) rather than the truth or falsity of story that determines the plot' (Abma, 1999: 171). There is a wealth of theoretical approaches to analysing oral and written data. Narrative researchers have been influenced by a number of social science methods for data analysis, including textual analysis, content analysis and discourse analysis. However, some authors are concerned to point out that narrative analysis is a loose, intuitive, artistic and poetic process and should not be viewed as formulaic, prefigured and narrow (Roberts, 2002). Baldwin (2004: 206) distinguishes narrative analysis from the analysis of narratives. This is a helpful distinction, in which he states that: 'The focus here is the dynamics of the narration and the process of production, treating narratives as facts in themselves, rather than the facts they contain.' Describing the sociology of stories, he speaks of the way in which a particular narrative seeks to empower or facilitate, degrade, control or dominate another. A researcher can bring together even incommensurable narratives to present several perspectives and/or a meta-analysis of phenomena, rather than simply analysing the content of a single narrative.

As one might expect there is no single method of narrative analysis. Some methods, however, are more formal than others. We will now look at some of the most common methods of narrative analysis in more detail.

Concepts related to narrative analysis

Sjuzet

Sjuzet is a term introduced by the Russian formalist critics to refer to the way in which the chronological raw materials of a story are organized. Cobley (2004: 243) notes that 'The story events which are to be *re*-presented by a narrative may have taken place, for example, within a particular chronological sequence; *sjuzet* can act to "rearrange" this sequence or ensure that the narration of some events is more extensive than others.'

Verisimilitude

Verisimilitude is defined as a logical and meaningful connection between described objects as opposed to a completely detailed analogue of them. In this sense textual coherence in context is more important than creating something real and related to readers' expectations of what is legitimate, believable and consonant. We mentioned the idea of truth telling in narrative research in Chapter 4, when we questioned the extent to which a person's story is real or is 'made up'.

Approaches to narrative analysis

Riessman (2006) identifies a number of approaches to narrative analysis which she classifies under the following headings:

- Thematic analysis
- Structural analysis
- Interactional analysis
- Performative analysis

Similarly Elliott (2005) argues that, to cope with the multiplicity of techniques included within the scope of narrative analysis, a typology (or classification) is required. She substantiates her argument by stating that a typology also has the benefit of explicating the methodological and epistemological differences that underpin the varying approaches to analysis. Elliott herself concentrates on content analysis, the analysis of structure and form and the social function of the narrative. Mishler (1995) also proposes a framework for understanding the numerous ways of analysing narratives, referring to meaning, structure and interaction. Braud and Anderson (1998) differentiate between content analysis, textual analysis, narrative analysis and discourse analysis, although they also see linkages and point out that each can complement the other. Overall, they argue, narrative analysis attempts to tell the story as the community or participants tell the story, following the story line and all its variants.

Lieblich et al. (1998) further typify narrative analysis as being not solely related to content or/and form, but also as being holistic or categorical. The first approach is a way of viewing the narrative in its completeness, the latter one that extracts smaller sections of text which can then be thematised or classified into categories. (This latter approach sounds similar to the practicalities of content analysis and thematic analysis, and will certainly be familiar to many nurse and healthcare researchers.)

The approach to narrative analysis is dependent upon a number of issues, but primarily on where the interest of the researcher lies, and of course the motivation for conducting narrative research in the first instance, i.e. the reason for the choice of method. The researcher might be more interested in the actual events, the experiences of the narrator, which form the content of the narrative – the 'what happened and why'. The differing approaches to narrative analysis can be undertaken simultaneously, complementing each other and deepening the under-standing of the data. This can be seen in the biographical–narrative–interpretive method of Chamberlayne et al. (2000), which clearly indicates a relationality between form, content and structure.

It could be argued that all narratives have a function; this may be taken into account when undertaking analyses of the text. So, for example, even when conducting content analysis, the function of the narrative might be seen to be the description of past and pre-sent events in order to explicate the meaning of those same events in the lives of the storyteller. Elliott (2005) calls this the 'evaluative function'.

Some researchers are predominantly interested in narrative form (the way in which a story is put together) and may seek out genres, metaphors, allegories in the text whilst simultaneously looking for coher-ence and context of both the narrative and the narrator (Box 8.1).

Thematic analysis

Roberts (2002) notes that in the process of analysis it becomes evid-ent that parts of the narrative are thematically connected. Aspects of the narrative are not drawn randomly, rather they are selected thematically. He states: 'This thematic field analysis approach involves a rigorous attention to hypothesis construction by careful reading of texts and an attempt to generate patterns' (Roberts, 2002: 121). Porter Abbott (2002) links thematic analysis (which is abstract) to repetition and interpretation (a concept closely aligned with analysis).

Content analysis

Content analysis can be applied either to single narratives or to a series of narratives. Where a single narrative is analysed (such as a biographical narrative or auto-ethnography), it is likely that it will be a holistic ana-lysis. Such an approach brings an awareness that is way beyond the individual, speaking also to sociological and cultural issues. Examples of holistic analysis of stories can be seen in Muncey's analysis of the deviant case in student nursing (and indeed her own auto-ethnography)

(Muncey, 2002) and McKenzie's narrative account of loss, 'singing into the void' (McKenzie, 2002: 22).

In the case of several narratives being analysed, the researcher will move from one story to the next, checking the main features; confirming previous accounts; identifying common elements; and developing a collective story. This would usually take place across a diverse range of cases, until some form of 'saturation' has been reached (though it does not go as far as grounded theory).

Structural analysis

Structural analysis focuses on the way in which the story is put together. The researcher is interested in how storytelling shapes the story and indeed the way it is conveyed by the narrator. Czarniawska (2004) describes structural analysis as an enterprise close to semiology and formalism. A well-known structural model of analysis comes from sociolinguists Labov and Waletzky (1967) as mentioned in Chapter 1. Based on the premise that narratives have formal structural properties and that patterns occur and recur, this structural model of narrative form identifies a number of elements that can be found in the text, namely an abstract, an orientation, a complicating action, an evaluative aspect, a resolution and a coda. Elliott (2005) is of the opinion that this structural model lends itself more to categorical analysis rather than to the holistic analysis of entire stories.

Interactional analysis

Elliott (2005: 38) links interactional analysis, which she describes as 'the interactional and institutional contexts in which narratives are produced, recounted and consumed', with the performance of the text.

Holistic and categorical analysis

In more detail, holistic analysts tend to work by identifying the narrative genre (for example, comedy or tragedy) or the direction (and intention) of the plot. This first approach can help the researcher to 'discern how the narrator wishes the events and experiences that are being recounted to be interpreted' (Elliott, 2005: 48). Gergen and Gergen (1987) write of this holistic analysis of the plot, referring to the way in which a story describes the ascent (progress), the decline (regress) and/or the stability of the narrator or characters.

Discourse analysis

Discourse analysis is a term used in the study of language; it draws upon a diversity of approaches and different epistemological foundations. In general it can be defined as a 'set of methods and theories for investigating language in use and language in contexts' (Wetherell et al., 2001: i). Hence, it can be applied to narrative, focusing on the use of language by the narrator to describe specific phenomena as well as being a way of understanding how the narrative might represent something of the dominant discourses.

Discourse analysis is an approach to research in its own right, drawing upon post-structuralist and postmodernist epistemologies and philosophies. However, it also has some practical application in the analysis of narrative texts.

Performative analysis

Performative analysis relates to how the narrative is communicated, the 'doing' of narrative. In this sense the researcher might be interested in how the narrative contributes to society, in other words, what is its action. Another term that could be used in this respect is narrative agency, which relates directly to the capacity of the narrative to cause events or engage in acts rather than merely report them.

Levels of analysis

Bakhtin (1981) conceives of a hierarchical relationship between discourses, which is similar to Shenhav's (2005: 75) suggestion that narrative analysis should take place on two levels: thick and thin levels. The thin level relates to 'events and situations described in a discourse and their order of appearance in the text', whereas the thick level of analysis relates to 'everything included in the "narration" and the relation between the components of the thin narrative'. Here he is drawing upon the work of Geertz (1973), who distinguishes between thick and thin description but clarifies that in thick description the relationship between content and process (and indeed the interactional aspect of the text) is viewed as central to the analytic process. Redman (2005) also differentiates between thick and thin narrative accounts, this in regard to the narrative formation of identity.

Analysis and interpretation

Narrative analysis and interpretation are intimately bound up, as they are in other qualitative research methods (Freshwater and Avis, 2004). This is most noticeable in the process of transcription, but occurs throughout the research process. In this sense Elliott (2005) recommends having an awareness of the variety of approaches to analysis before embarking on transcribing the data. Invariably throughout the process of analysis and interpretation, things are overlooked and things that are not there are added. We fill in the gaps, or, as Porter Abbott (2002) puts it, we 'overread' and 'underread'. This is not surprising: holding all the details of a story as we read it is difficult, and there are many aspects of books, research reports, newspapers and other texts that go unread. There are of course a number of vested personal, professional and cultural issues at play when we read. In overreading text, subtle qualities may be found in the story for which we have no direct evidence; these might include emotions and motives.

The most difficult thing to do when reading narratives is to stay in a state of uncertainty and avoid premature closure of the text. One example is the interpretation of the crux of the story. The way in which the crux is created, analysed and interpreted will impact the way in which the remainder of the narrative is analysed, although, of course, readings can also be re-read. Most people have had the experience of reading a book for the second time and finding it a very different experience, which begs the question, when does a narrative become another narrative?

Filling in the gaps is inevitable, for reading narrative is a 'tissue of insertions'. Interpreting narrative is also open to numerous approaches and methodological perspectives. Porter Abbott (2002) considers three fundamentally distinct means of interpreting narrative, these being intentional readings, symptomatic readings and adaptive readings.

Reflexivity

Narrative research as a whole demands a high level of reflexivity, not least in the process of analysis and interpretation of text, and the subsequent reporting of that process. It is important that researchers be open about and to the analytic process, reporting not only the narrative and plot, but also their own responses to it. Hence the boundaries between the narrative and the interpretation of that narrative are blurred. Hollway and Jefferson (2000) provide a number of practical prompts to facilitate a reflection on the process:

- What do you notice?
- Why do we notice what we notice?
- How can we interpret what we notice?
- How can we know that our interpretation is the right one?

Frank (2002) also provides some practical guidance about how to carry out narrative analysis, although not directly related to the project of reflexivity. He suggests that researchers:

- Take a sociological interest in the transcript, reading it firstly as a speech.
- Ask how the narrator marks the beginning and the end of the narrative; and how it is constructed.
- How is the narrator responding to questions, and in what manner?
- How does the narrator seek to affect the listener with the story; what change does the narrator seek to bring about in the listener?
- How/does the story represent a world view that is typical of some people in particular social situations, e.g. oppressed peoples?
- What larger societal narratives are embedded in the specific narratives told by the speaker?
- How are the social narratives being accepted or resisted?

Finally, although there are many different approaches to analysing text, Elliott (2005: 42) suggests that what unites methods of narrative analysis is the orientation to narrative, i.e. narrative is viewed as providing 'a relatively accurate description of events or experience through time'. Narrative is more than the sum of the parts. Ricoeur (1984), for example, suggests that the narrative must add up to something, that a narrative coherence exists. But that coherence is not necessarily about universality. Cobley (2004) states that narrative does not reveal universality; rather it has been instrumental in the promotion of difference, helping to preserve some memories and not others, and helping to ground some people in a given community and not others.

Summary

Narrative analysis is a complex and intense process, inextricably linked to the acts of interpretation and reflexivity. We have briefly outlined the main theoretical approaches to analysing narrative text, suggesting that the researcher does not need to stay firmly enmeshed in one particular approach. Rather the analytic and interpretive approach should be congruent with the aims and intended direction of the study, the researcher and of course the narrator. In this sense, narrative analysis can be as flexible or as rigid as the individual applying it.

9 Presenting Narrative Research

Authors who are involved in dissertation and thesis writing usually follow the main guidelines of their universities. Funding agencies sometimes have their own rules for writing up research, but most include the elements we will describe here.

Researchers are the sculptors of the final piece of writing, however much the input of the participants has helped shape the final version of the study. Although social science and nursing terminologies are part of the final account, narrative research needs to be written in an easy to read, narrative style. In other words, the researcher's report is a narrative that re-presents the stories of the participants' experience. The journey of discovery from listening to the participants' stories to presenting their experience in a narrative needs openness and honesty as well as language and narrative skills. This in itself can be problematic: the authors of a research account always choose from competing versions of meaning and interpretation. They have to judge which words or phrases best present the phenomenon; this means making choices based on subjectivity, and this subjectivity must be acknowledged. Wolcott (2001) advises an early start with writing as many of us forget details which we haven't written down. This technique is also useful for clarifying one's thoughts. The final narrative will not overwhelm the authors if many important elements have already been written up beforehand. Writers do, however, refine their writing in an ongoing process of thinking, data collection, analysis and reflection. Finally, though, the meaning that the participants give to their experience, and the context on which it is based, must be captured, and the writer's narrative must resonate in the reader and give a sense of location. Writing is never neutral; it has political and ideological elements and reflects the subjectivity and the personal location of the researcher as well as that of the participants. Denzin (2001: 23) declares more than once that 'Writing is not an innocent practice. We know the world only through our representations of it.'

The experience of the participants in research is storied, but 'the meaning making process of the researcher is also storied' (Gudmundsdottir, 1998) and thus becomes re-telling. Readers should be able to locate themselves in the researcher's position while reading the story but also hear the participants and empathise with them. The writer has his or her own intentions, which others might recognise, but readers of the final account also have their own perspectives that influence their understanding. All are affected by the culture in which they live and the final account resonates with the feelings and beliefs of that culture. The ideas in the write-up are jointly owned by the writer and the participants.

Merely retelling the stories does not suffice. The narrative is an analysis of the stories told by those involved and includes the development, modification and creation of theories. It describes the meaning of the phenomenon under study and its essential core. Ultimately the researcher achieves a transformation of the data received from participants, and the work includes his or her own description and interpretation; thus a researcher's narrative is never just an attempt to represent the voices of the participants: the writer is not a 'ventriloquist' (a term sometimes used in poetry). There is, of course, an obligation on the part of the researcher to be mindful of the words and thoughts of the participants (Holloway, 2005) and to contextualise them in time and place. Not to take this into account could be considered unethical.

Presenting the narrative

Writing up narrative research is not easy and is a lonely task for a single researcher. It is different from a conventional thesis or dissertation which becomes a 'rite de passage' (Noy, 2003), written in traditional style and similar for most postgraduates. Of course, research accounts need the requisite and appropriate number of steps, but the narrative in this type of research often takes a different form. There are several differences. While in quantitative inquiry researchers generally – though not always – adopt a neutral stance demonstrated by the passive voice, and the use of terms such as 'the author', and 'the researcher', qualitative researchers acknowledge and demonstrate their active involvement and responsibility for what is written in the completed text. Language and style express the intentions of the researchers and highlight their priorities.

Most – though not all – qualitative researchers present a full written account or report at the completion of their project, and the exact form it takes depends on the type of research. Different types of text have to be constructed for different readerships or audiences. The writer is the mediator between the participants and the readers; thus the account is a mediation process. The ethnographer Van Maanen (1988) suggests three different possibilities for telling the tale or presenting the text: realist, confessional and impressionistic. The realist description is factual and objective, usually written in the third person, while the confessional tale includes subjective and personal elements and is concerned with the author's own experiences before and during the research process. It is reflective and reflexive, and presented in the first person, and prior assumptions are uncovered. The impressionist description portrays the phenomenon or the participants' experiences in an interesting way almost like a novel, though it is not an invention.

In good narrative research the reader will find elements of all three types of tale. The rationale, literature review and methodology – including an audit trail – are by nature factual descriptions although they too are mindful of the research participants and the writer in the tale. The narrative needs coherence and flow to be convincing. Researchers writing a PhD thesis or a report for a funding agency also need a clear description of the research process itself, including an audit trail; hence the final account always suffers from being fractured in some sections. The final writings of different authors are diverse because of the nature of the phenomena under study in narrative research; hence a great variety of ways of writing up exist in this type of research. It is less rule governed and does not always have the same format. Atkinson et al. (2003: 171) confirm that much diversity exists in the reports of qualitative research 'encompassing different disciplinary styles, textual conventions and subject matter'. Narrative research is no exception, and variety of presentation is permissible as long as the researcher fulfils the purpose of the study.

Narrative inquiry is often more distrusted than other types of research as it relies on stories which might be seen as unreliable and not 'the truth', and on the rhetoric of the author of the final account which might be seen as 'journalistic'. We have explained, however, that the perceptions of the participants differ from but are as important as factual data. There are elements of good journalism contained in the narrative write-up, such as its rhetoric – that of persuasion, opinion and ornamentation – but it also needs to be scientific, with reason, logic, methods and evidence (Coffey et al., 1996: 4).

The elements of the report and the process of writing

What does a write-up include? Some sections such as the rationale and the methodology will contain elements similar to other research reports, be they quantitative or qualitative. These are routine elements of most research reports, although narrative researchers occasionally present them in different forms. Writers also have to define the terms and concepts they use, either when they are first mentioned or in a *glossary* at the beginning or end of the research. The explanation should not be a dictionary definition but one that has specific meaning in the area under study and is used in textbooks on methodology or topic.

In narrative research in particular, writers need to develop a good *title* (see Chapter 12). A title can set the scene for the whole of the report and arouse interest in the reader. Some examples are as follows:

Challenging 'ordinary' pain: narratives of people who live with pain (Becker, 2001)

Narrative representations of chronic illness experience: cultural models of illness, mind, and body in stories concerning the temporomandibular joint (Garro, 1994)

Recovering bodies: illness, disability and life writing (Couser, 1997)

The *abstract* is a summary of the research including a short description of the topic, the aim, the methodology including design and approach, procedures and sample. A summary of the main findings is also given.

Usually the tale proceeds in the following way:

(1) Authors explain the background of the study, give a rationale for the research, and describe the setting and context in which it takes place (introduction).
(2) They describe and evaluate what others have found while exploring the same phenomenon and point to the gap in the state of knowledge and show how they plug the gap (literature review).
(3) They describe and justify the approaches and strategies they adopted to investigate the phenomenon they wished to research (research design which includes methodology and strategies).
(4) They describe what they found (findings).
(5) They interpret the findings, set out their arguments and enter into a dialogue with the literature which confirmed or challenged what they found (discussion).
(6) They tell the reader what they have learnt from their research (conclusion).
(7) They describe its significance for professional or academic practice (implications).
(8) They reflect on the journey that they have taken as researchers (reflexivity and reflectivity).

The introduction

The introduction is one of the most important elements in the research as it sets the scene for the researcher's narrative. Writers start by pulling the reader into the text through an interesting discussion of the *context, importance* and *scope* of the research. However, the main aim of the introduction is to state the *rationale*, i.e. the reasons for the research and the way the research question or problem has been developed. Usually this includes the reasons why the writer found the topic interesting and unusual, why the research has been necessary, and how and why it will be significant for clinical practice (even though this should become obvious in the process of the narrative).

The place of the literature

In narrative inquiry, as in other types of qualitative research, the literature relevant to the study is used in different ways from a conventional literature review. In quantitative research the review is usually a survey of all the major literature available on the topic under study, while in qualitative research it is initially an overview of the main areas of the research and shows that the aim or purpose of the inquiry really fills a gap in knowledge.

The initial literature review

The initial review of the literature should take account of the nature of narrative research and show that the writers did not let themselves be forced into specific areas of the study. Silverman (2005: 300) states that a literature review should demonstrate both knowledge and critical thinking and contribute to the wider debate of the topic area. This means that the exploration of the literature is not mere description but a critical analysis of that which has gone on before in the research about the topic or phenomenon. A good, clear overview of the literature provides context and frame, linking the research to the writing and researching of others who have explored the same or a similar topic. Most writers divide this into relevant sections of the area to be investigated and the issues that need highlighting. Although many writers state the main aim of the research at its very beginning, it can only be fully obvious at the end of the literature overview.

The in-depth literature review

The in-depth literature review should be carried out during and after the data analysis, and is ongoing from the beginning to the completion of the researcher's narrative. It will later provide a dialogue with the major findings from the data and contribute to the process of exploration. In the initial literature review the writer poses an interesting problem for the reader so that the following chapters seem like detective work to reach the solution of the problem. In the ongoing in-depth literature review, however, the researcher who has analysed the participants' narratives ties the literature to the themes that emerged. For instance, if participants tell their stories of chronic illness and the reaction of others to it, the researcher might generate the theme 'the experience of stigma'. She or he then ties this theme to the existing literature about similar research in which people have experienced being negatively labelled. The discussion of the literature demands that the researcher actively engages in the debate, understands arguments, reads critically, and evaluates others' way of thinking about the theme.

The research design

The researcher needs to state the delimitations and limitations of the research. *Delimitations* are the boundaries which determine the scope of a study and sample. *Limitations* are restrictions or shortcomings of the research. Some of these are a result of the decisions of the researcher; others are generated by circumstances over which the researcher has no control.

The methodology, methods and strategies

The initial plan of the research has to be described, and also how and why the researchers deviated from it. They show the *methodological framework* and the *strategies, tools and techniques* they used in their approach. A detailed description of the data collection and analysis will help the reader to follow the audit trail. The writers also show why they have discarded alternative types of inquiry and chosen the specific method and strategies adopted.

The write-up justifies the choice of narrative approach and the detailed steps in the research process such as selection of sample, collection and analysis of data as well as examples from these phases of research. This part also includes a demonstration of *trustworthiness* or 'validity' of the research (discussed in Chapter 10). Writers usually disclose what they did and how they did it, but they sometimes forget to explain why they chose the approach from a list of possible alternatives. On the other hand, they sometimes give a lengthy – though unnecessary – description of alternative strategies that they might have taken. The history of the research is important, however, as narrative inquiry rarely follows a linear path. Indeed in this type of study the focus might change in the process, and the researcher must justify this and make it explicit.

The description of the initial *sampling* plan explains how the researchers gained access to the participants, and how many people were included and why. Exclusion criteria are also stated: for instance, why were some potential participants excluded from the study?

It is difficult to write up the methodology and procedures but explanations and descriptions of are necessary so that readers can understand the narrative and trace the audit trail.

Findings and discussion

In this section, the author shows the links between the findings and the data that was collected and analysed. There are two choices for presenting this part of the writing up. Writers may use the traditional way of presenting the findings, by giving a straight description and including examples and relevant quotes from participants. Alternatively, writers may combine the findings and discussion. Whatever the writer decides, the major findings which had been developed into themes need to be linked to the existing, relevant literature, including both early, seminal writing and up-to-date references. The critical dialogue with the literature will provide part of the researcher's narrative. This will not only contain the 'first order concepts' of the participants but also the interpretation of the data by the researcher who transformed the data in the process of analysis. The *theoretical framework* which has been developed during the process of the research is presented throughout the description of findings and the discussion.

Most researchers add a *reflective chapter* or section towards the end of their study in which they reflect on the process of the research, their relationship with the participants and other issues that they found intriguing or problematic although, increasingly, reflections are inserted throughout and are central to the study. The limitations of the research can also be discussed here. This gives the reader an insight into the researcher's thinking and deliberation and describes the researcher's roles and journey.

Conclusion and implications for practice

Narrative inquiry results in learning about the meaning that the participants attribute to their experience which is in its turn interpreted by the researcher. In the conclusion writers need to demonstrate the claim that they make in relation to the aim of the research and what they found out through completing it. They make explicit what they learnt, mainly the knowledge they acquired through carrying out the research, but do not at this stage introduce new ideas though they can point the way to future research. Wolcott (2001) argues that the conclusion may open up new questions generated by the research. The conclusion is solely about these issues and the writer does not introduce any new literature which had not been previously discussed.

In the section on *implications* the writer shows how the research might enhance and improve clinical practice. It points to solutions of problems in the practice settings. Creswell (2003: 149) expresses it very clearly and states that there should be:

- Several ways in which the study adds to knowledge in the field
- Some ideas on how the research can help enhance practice
- Reasons why the research will improve policies or practices

Implications relate directly to the conclusions of the study and what has been learnt in the process of the specific research and not to the findings of other researchers.

The use of quotes and examples

When discussing the findings, extracts from the stories of the participants demonstrate that the interpretation and conclusions drawn from the research are appropriate. Qualitative researchers try to make their arguments credible to readers by using quotes from participants as well as summarising their stories. Quotes can precede or follow the researcher's summaries, descriptions and interpretations. In narrative inquiry these sections from stories and interview answers might be extensive, more so than in other qualitative research – although a report consisting mainly of quotes or strings of quotes when the researcher attempts to present an argument or to make a point is not acceptable. The selection of these quotes relies on the judgement of the researchers and their interpretation of the meaning that the participants attribute to events and happenings in their lives. The quote or quotes (a single quote is not always enough) illustrate the finding and argument and are directly related to it. In most approaches quotes confirm patterns discovered through the research and demonstrate the feelings and thoughts of the majority of participants, but in narrative inquiry unique ideas of an individual can also be described and illustrated by their own words. Quotes provide evidence for some of the statements and interpretations that the researcher has made. They also enliven the story and make it more convincing. At other times they point to a unique perception of the phenomenon by an individual or to a 'deviant case'. Though quotes are anonymous and not attributable to a specific, named individual, an identifier (for instance, participant 3, practice nurse B, consultant X, Dr A) or a pseudonym can be given. A specific name (which must be a pseudonym) rather than a number or letter makes a narrative study more interesting and lively and less like a report. The identifier ensures that the quotes throughout the study are not just taken from the words of one or two participants who are articulate and whose words make a dramatic impact on the reader. It also shows that the writer does not over-identify with just a few people in the study and neglects the ideas of other participants. Great care must be taken that individuals cannot be identified by their quotes. The writer selects the quotes judiciously as inappropriate choices can mislead the reader. Truthful representation of what the researcher understands from the data about the participants' thoughts and feelings is important. (See also Chapter 13.)

We summarise some of the reasons that White et al. (2003: 313) give for the use of quotes:

- They show the participants' use of language, concepts and expressions in the discussion of a phenomenon
- They give the meaning people attribute to the area, topic or phenomenon under study
- They point to the stance of participants towards the research topic
- They illustrate the depth, richness and diversity of people's stories

These quotes, so White et al. advise, should also contribute to and extend the text rather than just repeating an argument the researcher has made, hence they need explanation and interpretation. Of course, the writer contextualises the quotes, and comments on and engages with them. Writers can also enhance the text and make it more credible and vivid by examples or vignettes. Examples and vignettes might enhance the text, act as tools for illustration and provide more immediacy.

Mason (2002) observes that the presentation of the research needs convincing academic arguments. These are constructed by the researcher to persuade the reader that the research was justified and its outcome the result of an appropriate analysis of the data. These arguments should relate to the aim of the research and must be presented clearly to make them accessible to the reader.

Contextualisation and 'thick description'

Contextualisation gives coherence to the writing and shows that narrative inquiry unlike laboratory research does not happen in a vacuum. It locates both writer and participants in their context: time and the physical and social environment. Thick description (Geertz, 1973), a term often used in all types of qualitative research and important especially in narrative inquiry, means the use of detailed and intensive portrayals of the characters in the study, their social world and experiences. It is now common that writers acknowledge their own location, background and influences to uncover their subjectivity and show that they are not objective and neutral; for instance, critical care nurses would acknowledge their own stance and location in nursing when they carry out narrative research in the field.

Although all the elements of the research story, be it in a report, a dissertation or an article, are necessary, the writer also takes into account the language itself as well as its aesthetic and communicative power achieved through imagination, hard work and skillful use of metaphors. The reader, however, must know what the author's narrative is all about and hence it must have cohesion, clarity and plausibility.

The writing-up needs both 'grab and good science' (Gilgun, 2005), meaning that it gives the participant's story in a vivid and interesting way as well as conveying the theoretical and more abstract ideas of the researcher. The writer's story resembles that of the participant in the sense that it has a beginning, a middle and an end, but it is generally better organised and follows a logical path.

One of the criticisms writers make (Wolcott, 2001; Jones, 2005a) is about the conventionality and routine presentation of research reports which often leaves out a discussion of the researcher's relationship with the participants. The final narrative includes elements of the identities of both researcher and participant.

Performative social science

Writing a text is not the only way to present the narrative from participants' stories. Kip Jones claims that we live in a performance culture (see on-line newsgroup, Perform Soc Sci, 2006), and researchers even 'perform' when they write or orally and visually present their research. Jones argues for innovation in presenting narrative research. The creative tension between the social science involved and artistic elements, between the reality of facts and the reality of feelings and thoughts (Coffey et al., 1996), enhances the research. The creator generates not just words but also images and pictures for the reader. Even spaces in the writing, or indications of silence, are significant. Researchers might wish to demonstrate the findings through poetry, pictures, drawings or photographs, or through drama. This is a fairly recent way of developing and presenting narrative research, and can be interesting and rewarding though many universities are not yet ready to accept this in a PhD thesis. This presentation, of course, differs from writing text as the participants become characters in a play. Many researchers believe that performance reflects more closely the character of narrative research than a dry, routine piece of writing. Indeed, this way of presenting the research is sometimes used to teach health professionals about their clients' emotions and problems. Keen and Todres (2006) give examples of research based theatre. Stage plays were performed in front of audiences of health professionals and these examples showed that much was learnt from these productions.

Performance based narrative work is located between art and science. Jones (2005b) stresses the importance of knowledge transfer and the need for new ways to disseminate findings. We would argue that this could attract a new audience for narrative research as well as refreshing the perspective of traditional academics and professionals. Jones claims that the possibilities in this arena are endless and include the visual arts as well as poetry and the new media. The complexity of narrative inquiry might be reflected in these innovative ways. For novice researchers this may be unsafe as it sometimes defies university regulations and might be misunderstood by funding bodies. Experienced researchers, however, might persuade others more easily that presentations in novel ways are appropriate and exciting while at the same time conveying the knowledge that has been captured through the research. Saldaña (2003) speaks of dramatising data, which may be done through role play or theatre. He writes of participants as characters on a stage, but much of what he says is also helpful in writing a research narrative. We will here give some of his suggestions. The researcher should examine:

(1) The participants' ('players' in Saldaña's writing) perspectives on their lives.
(2) What they do to achieve their aims and objectives.
(3) The perceptions and interventions of others.
(4) Their own perspectives on the experience of the participants.
(5) The evaluation and comments generated by the experience of everyday life.

(adapted from Saldaña, 2003: 221).

Complexity

It is almost inevitable that the final narrative or account of the researcher is a simplification as the participants live in their own complex world that they seek to describe and which can never wholly be grasped by the researcher. Considering the breadth and depth of the material acquired, the writing cannot be comprehensive and include every thought and feeling of others. Wengraf (2000) does, however, stress the need for quality in 'condensed representation' of the rich data. This also includes the complex and sometimes expert knowledge of the researchers themselves, be it methodological or nursing specific. They bring complexity to the story because they transcend the stories of the participants; in other words, raw data are accepted, rejected, transformed and interpreted throughout the study and especially in the final presentation.

Conclusion

Writers also discuss questions of authenticity and usefulness of qualitative research outcomes. Entertaining the readership and creating immediacy and interest are not enough. However, if the writer can give an interesting account which includes affective and aesthetic elements as well as truthfulness and clarity, the writing becomes readable and useful because it can be grasped by the reader. Disseminating the findings to others is, after all, the main aim of the researcher-writer.

Morse and Richards (2002) claim that thinking about a qualitative project goes beyond completion of the research. This applies to narrative inquiry where ideas are continuously developed. New stories are being told every day to professionals and researchers in the clinical arena, hence the researcher never truly finishes the research project.

Summary

The procedures for the final account are to some extent in the control of researchers. They do, however, have to follow the procedures and processes that their universities or grant-giving bodies demand from them, unless they can negotiate different forms of presentation. At the centre, however, are the quality of the account and the re-presentation of the participants' stories in a clear and evocative way. The account of the researcher should be scientifically sound and communicative, and have aesthetic value.

Critical Issues

10 Trustworthiness and Authenticity in Narrative Research

In all types of inquiry, researchers attempt to be trustworthy and honest – unless they set out to deceive. Qualitative researchers, too, are concerned with the trustworthiness and authenticity of their accounts by presenting the reality of the participants. It is important to recognise, however, that there are two different levels on which to discuss authenticity (or validity) in narrative inquiry: the original story of the participants, as well as the narrative in which the researcher re-presents their stories; not only do participants tell stories but the account of the researcher who carries out narrative inquiry is also a narration.

The participant's story

Researchers hope that the stories of the participants are true. They do know, however, that narrators sometimes have bad memories, are muddled, or overdramatise for effect. Plausibility and even credibility do not suffice in narrative research; after all, novelists and fraudsters alike tell plausible stories persuading the listener that they speak the truth. Narrators sometimes make mistakes, and occasionally they tell deliberate lies. The narrative researcher takes this into account. Lying deliberately or unconsciously does not mean necessarily that there is no truth in the story. Of course the stories may be fiction, but fiction too can illustrate reality, and the illustration depends on how the stories are told. Even when lying, storytellers illuminate aspects of their world because they lie for a reason. Sometimes, though not always, researchers recognise this. Sandelowski (1996) quotes the Personal Narratives Group (1989: 261) 'Unlike the reassuring Truth [*their* capitalisation] of the scientific idea, the truths of narratives are neither open to proof nor self-evident.' This does not mean, however, that participants usually tell untruths. As long as they identify with the ideas they present, the researcher can develop knowledge from the stories they bring to the inquiry. They describe their world and their reality as they see it – from their perspective. This includes, of course, the basis of their stories in temporal and cultural elements. Thus, although individuals give their own unique, individual view, it is not 'merely' that but embedded in time and culture (see Chapter 1). By telling their story in context, individuals offer 'knowledge about much more than themselves' (Sandelowski, 1996: 119). Researchers do trust the people they study even if they can't 'verify' the 'truths' of their stories.

Example
A patient might tell her story of a hospital stay. She firmly believes in a system that is free at the point of uptake, and values the setting and situation as the best that is available on limited funds. This story sounds different from that of a person who believes in a private care system and demonstrates all the faults that a publicly funded system might have. Both stories are true but depend upon the beliefs and ideology of patients. Neither story is necessarily a reflection of 'objective reality'.

Qualitative researchers such as Lincoln and Guba (1985) suggest a member check to find out whether the interviews represent the 'true story' of the participant. This means the transcript or a summary of the interview is sent back to the participant. In narrative inquiry this is inappropriate for several reasons (phenomenologists in particular disagree with member checks). First of all, the written text is not the original as it was first conceived but a 'different form of discourse', according to Czarniawska (2004), and it offers a different and less direct perspective. She states that the participant usually sees it as a written text and corrects or retells it accordingly, locating it in a different frame of reference. Also, the researcher and the narrator have co-created the story in interaction with each other, and the written text does not wholly reflect this. The full research account is a transformation by the researcher of what he or she receives from the participant, and it usually focuses on the phenomenon under study rather than the participants. Sandelowski (1996) argues that research conventions may prevent the participants from recognising their stories because of this transformation. The re-presentation in a scholarly vein – as good science – takes a different form from the original telling of the story. The research agenda too differs from the agenda of the participant. Although the researcher's narrative has to be faithful to the participant's account, it also transcends it. Sandelowski speaks of the 'revisionist nature of narratives' (p. 119). The story might be understood by the researcher's academic peers as a 'good' piece of research but misread by the participants who will not always be able to understand the form of language used in the researcher's account.

Most of the writers who discuss the trustworthiness of accounts, be they the participants' or the researchers', stress that the insider's interpretation is no more true than that of the outsider, but the researcher has the last word by imposing his or her researcher perspective on the interview or observation. Bryman (2001), too, sums up the problematics of member checking. He claims that researchers write for a readership of scholars and peers. This means that they always take the research to the level of developing concepts, an 'etic' view, which includes but also goes beyond the participants' perspectives. The researchers must describe in some depth how their interpretations of the stories' contents differ from those of the participants.

The narrative of the researcher

The researcher's narrative is more than just the story of the participant. Yes, it re-presents the voice of the person who has taken part in the research, but the narrative can be recognised by the academic community as such and is not merely the retelling of the participant's story. Researchers transform and interpret the story. Indeed Phillips (1997: 104) states that he sees the researcher as just a 'scribe' if he or she merely retells the stories which participants generate and takes them as evidence without critical reflection. Phillips observes that researchers may be more interested in a dramatic and interesting story than in the 'truth'. This may mean a strong temptation to write something that illustrates their points and should be resisted.

Bruner (1986) claims that narratives are not necessarily testable and verifiable facts but instead plausible and dramatic versions of experience. Unfortunately, that which is measurable and generalisable is often seen as more valid in research. He also maintains that the truth of narratives can't be established through falsification like other research processes but can only approach 'verisimilitude' (1991), that is, something that appears to be the truth but cannot be proven. This term has been used by social science earlier. Verisimilitude, however – a term also used by Polkinghorne (1988), is not enough.

Research knowledge acquired through participant narratives is provisional, meaning that it may be true for now, this moment, for here, for this locality and this culture. The truth cannot be absolute, certain and forever. Of course, the 'truth' of the researcher's narrative is occasionally in conflict with the story of the participants. Phillips maintains that the researcher's perspective alone does not necessarily have 'authoritative status', but neither do the stories of the participants.

Subjectivity, objectivity and intersubjectivity

There is a distinction between objective and subjective elements of truth. If researchers want to explore what experience means for participants – if nurses wish to know what their condition or treatment or care means for their patients – they are more interested in the subjective aspects of truth, indeed subjectivity becomes a resource for researchers, be it the subjectivity of those being interviewed or the researcher's own. Bias is a prejudice or an unfair influence which prevents researchers from considering certain factors or problems which might not fit their world view. Narrative researchers don't often use this term and instead speak of subjectivity. Any researcher has 'biases', assumptions and prejudices that might prevent him or her from acting 'objectively'. Researchers have to disclose to the readers of the research where they stand, and how their own subjectivity has influenced the study. Their own experience of the setting and situation might generate ideas which could be accepted after the research, or rejected because the inquiry itself did not confirm them.

Only recently has subjectivity officially been accepted in academic writing and research. Stories offer a subjective perspective on experienced reality, and hence they have to be evaluated in a different way from other types of data. Human beings tell their stories in a personal, subjective manner. Subjectivity used to be seen as a problem of qualitative research, while quantitative inquiry seemed to be requiring 'objectivity' and a neutral stance. However, even in quantitative research this is debated. All research has elements of subjectivity; even natural science research depends on the choices of the researcher in the focus, selection and interpretation of data.

The subjective element is inherent in the main source of narrative data though even people's stories and those of researchers are never wholly subjective as they are based in their culture and time. However, this subjectivity means that participants claim that their stories are true, and indeed the researcher has to believe that they are authentic. This 'truth' is not always congruent with factual or historical truth as people make individual judgements about their experiences. Nevertheless, this does not mean historical and subjective truths contradict each other. Both are equally authentic; indeed, Kikuchi and Simmons (1996) go even further than this and claim that two distinct and different stories about the same condition could both be accepted as true. There might be several versions of social reality. The creative story can illuminate the nature of truth, although it may not correspond to fact or 'objective reality' which in itself is a problematic concept. Winter states (though in a different context) that this correspondence of truth and facts is merely 'a claim, rather than an objective criterion for judgement' (Winter, 2002: 144). Also, the researcher isn't necessarily interested in facts but in the perspective of the participants and how they reflect on their motivations, how they justify their actions, and how they give meaning to their experience. Altheide and Johnson (1994) also claim that objectivity is not possible. Knowledge is 'perspectival' and interpretive, depending on the stance of those who find, explore and develop it. Therefore the processes by which the researcher gained this knowledge have to be made explicit and transparent for others.

Qualitative researchers often recognise whether stories are authentic or not, because of the elements of intersubjectivity and *Verstehen*. They acknowledge the mutuality and reciprocity in the human condition and empathetically recognise the aspects of universality in the perspectives of others; some of their own experiences resonate with those of the participants and increase understanding. Reciprocity also demands a reflection on issues of power and equality. In narrative inquiry the issue of power is, of course, important, but as the participants have much control over the way they wish to tell their stories, the power of the researcher has not the same constraining effect as in other types of qualitative study.

Moustakas (1994) uses the term 'intersubjective truth'. He suggests that according to Husserl 'each can experience and know the other, not exactly as one experiences and knows oneself but in the sense of empathy and copresence' (p. 57). This idea can be developed: truth is based in the unique perspective of individuals and their self-knowledge. They share the world with others, communicate with them and develop intersubjective understanding. The researchers too are part of this world, and this assists them in understanding it and grasping other people's views as well as the essence of the phenomenon under study. This form of 'validity' is similar to the ideas about ontological authenticity described by Guba and Lincoln (1989) and linked to that of 'thick description' by Geertz (1973), which we will discuss later.

There is also the 'words and deeds' debate: Do people do what they claim to do? Atkinson et al. (2003) observe that 'action' consists not only of 'observed doings' but also of spoken words. These authors debate ideas of Dean and Whyte (1958) who suggest that the discussion should centre not on words and deeds but on what participants uncover about their perspectives rather than the 'factual truth'. These go through the filter of culture and participant motive; hence competing accounts may exist of the same event. Atkinson et al. advise, for instance, that researchers examine the participants' accounts and the linguistic devices they use in their stories, be they 'hedging' or direct telling, etc., as well as underlying motives in a specific cultural context. Hence these writers maintain that objectivity and 'truth' are problematic and by no means simple. Roberts (2002) also discusses the issue that stories have a different kind of credibility, to do with imagination and psychological truth, and uncover a depth that factual accounts don't have.

Narrative as science and art: plausibility and rigour

The artistic quality of narrative inquiry has already been discussed. Artistic works need to be plausible and persuasive so that the viewer/reader has a faithful portrait of the meaning the 'artist' wants to create. If this is successful, the research has credibility and fidelity.

Narrative research, however, is also social science. This means it needs structure, consistency and coherence. Science, in fact, demands rigour: Sandelowski (1986) advises researchers to have rigour. However, in a later article she speaks of 'rigor or rigor mortis' [*sic*], stating that the term is problematic and might imply inflexibility (Sandelowski, 1993: 27). She believes that this rigidity endangers creativity and the search for meaning. Of course, the way researchers define rigour is important. Generally the term is applied in quantitative research and implies exactness, measurability, validity and clear standards. In qualitative research it can be related to coherence, consistency and contextualisation. Researchers need to be mindful of this but also faithful to the participants' ideas and feelings. Narrative research in particular is based on trust between researcher and participants, as the latter will only disclose their thoughts and emotions if a relationship has been established. Davies and Dodd (2002) believe that rigour is closely linked to ethics, in particular, because ethical behaviour includes disclosure of the researcher's location in the research process. Researchers are accountable for the way they ask questions and the way they report the accounts of the participants. They need to make visible their decision-making processes and show them to be ethical and rigorous.

Reflexivity and contextuality

In narrative research, as in other types of qualitative inquiry, reflexivity is a necessary element of quality and assists in establishing the trustworthiness of the study. It means thoughtfulness and reflection on their relationship with the participants and their own reactions towards them. The researchers not only consider carefully the participants' narratives – including emotions and meanings – but also their own stance, location and feelings. They need to explore their own assumptions and how these have influenced the research. To be considered trustworthy, the research is shown to uncover the researcher's own interests and background, and how these influenced the research strategies and procedures. Researchers need to be aware of the contextual as well as the holistic character of narrative inquiry, and reflective about the many influences on the participants and the research process of a narrative study.

Research knowledge, as most other knowledge, is provisional, meaning that it might be true for now, for here, for a particular individual. It can never be absolute, certain and once-and-forever truth. Perhaps we need a new and different vocabulary to establish quality in narrative research. It might be better to talk of trustworthiness, credibility and authenticity as criteria for quality rather than truth; this is what Lincoln and Guba (1985; and see Guba and Lincoln, 1989) suggest. The concept of validity, however, is still used in narrative research, particularly in phenomenological studies, though the meaning of validity here is quite different and less precise.

The question of validity

The traditional criteria for research are validity and reliability. Narrative researchers often find these concepts inappropriate; however, they cannot opt out of this discussion. Narrative inquiry is one of the approaches within qualitative research, and its quality has to be judged by some of the criteria that apply to the latter. We have discussed the notion of truth which is after all another word for validity. Validity is a term used in quantitative research, and Bryman (2001) claims that we cannot simply apply the same criterion to qualitative inquiry.

Some writers argue for the retention of the criteria for validity and reliability (Maxwell, 2004; Silverman, 2005) but agree that these have a different meaning when applied to qualitative research. Others such as Wolcott (1994) and Stake (1995) reject these criteria as inappropriate and believe that each research project is unique and needs contextuality. Sparkes (2001) asserts that qualitative researchers do not agree about these terms or criteria, and that there is no shared understanding of validity. All these authors criticise the obsession with validity.

Reliability and contextualisation

Findings are reliable if the research tool has been consistent and if they are replicable, that is, if the study can be repeated and produces the same results in similar circumstances and under similar conditions. Obviously, narrative research cannot ever be repeated. Not only are the stories of the participants unique (though embedded in their culture) but the researcher, as the research instrument, will also affect the research through his or her specific and individual perspective, background and characteristics. As this research is contextual and often even context dependent, a similar study may well generate different results. Dahlberg et al. (2001) claim that internal contradictions in the research report might make the research less credible and valid.

More usually the terms of trustworthiness and authenticity are utilised. Lincoln and Guba (1985, and see Guba and Lincoln, 1989) popularised these concepts and claim these as the standard for qualitative research and thereby they 'reconceptualise' validity (Smith, 1998). Lincoln and Guba saw trustworthiness as methodological soundness and adequacy which was achieved through developing dependability, credibility, transferability and confirmability.

(1) *Dependability*. If a study, that is the narrative of the researcher, is dependable, it should be consistent and accurate. Its adequacy can be judged by the reader through the clarity of the decision-making process in an audit trail in which the researcher describes in detail the research design, data collection and analysis as well as the way he or she arrived at the conclusion.

(2) *Credibility*. Credibility has a similar meaning to internal validity. Internal validity is of particular importance in narrative research. It confirms the extent to which the researcher re-presents the social reality of the participants and the meanings they give to their experiences. The reader should feel that the account is plausible and recognise its credibility. Of course, credibility is not enough (this will be discussed later).

(3) *Transferability*. Lincoln and Guba suggest that the findings in a particular context are transferable to similar situations with similar types of participant. Knowledge and theory that are developed should be relevant and applicable in other settings. It is necessary, however, that these settings have a related context as the 'context stripping' of quantitative research is not appropriate for qualitative inquiry. In narrative research in particular, context is crucial.

(4) *Confirmability*. The reader can evaluate the research by the way in which findings and conclusions achieve the aim of the study and are not the result of the researcher's prior assumptions and preconceptions. Again, this needs transparency in the audit trail. Readers can recognise how researchers arrived at the findings and the meaning of the participants' stories. For this knowledge of context, background and feelings of the researcher should be open to public scrutiny. Dahlberg et al. (2001) ask for clarity and intellectual honesty but they also advise sensitivity to the phenomenon or phenomena under study.

Lincoln and Guba and others after them developed checklists and criteria by which the trustworthiness of qualitative studies could be established. We have already mentioned member check (which is problematic) and audit trail. Added to this is 'peer debriefing' when colleagues analyse the data, and their findings are compared with those of the researcher. Their overlap or similarity demonstrates that the ideas of the participants are represented. Triangulation is another technique for establishing trustworthiness. Methodological triangulation, which means the use of more than one approach to the study, is not appropriate in narrative research where the participant narratives are the only data sources. Barbour (2003) criticises the overuse of checklists in qualitative research. We suggest that in narrative inquiry they are even more inappropriate, though Barbour quotes Seale (1999) who maintains that the checklist can be used as an *aide-mémoire* that makes the researchers aware of their own practices. Criteria can be useful as there has to be a standard for 'good' qualitative research; Barbour, however, does take issue with 'technical essentialism' which means overuse of detailed checklists.

As important as the notion of trustworthiness is that of authenticity which Guba and Lincoln add in 1989 (as described by Holloway and Wheeler, 2002). Authenticity includes the following:

(1) *Fairness*. The researcher must be fair and just to participants and take their social context into account. Informed consent is gained throughout and not just at the beginning of the study.
(2) *Ontological authenticity*. This means that those involved will have been helped to understand their social world and their human condition through the research.
(3) *Educative authenticity*. Through intersubjective understanding, participants improve their understanding of others.
(4) *Catalytic authenticity*. Decision-making by participants should be enhanced by the research.
(5) *Tactical authenticity*. The research should empower participants.

A study is authentic when the process is adequate, when the ideas of the participants are appropriately presented and when participants and readers have better insight into their own problems and can improve their situation (Erlandson et al., 1993).

Transferability or generalisability

Generally we utilise restricted and narrow notions of generalisability. Regardless of the assurances of Lincoln and Guba that transferability is a more suitable word than generalisability, there is still a strong feeling in the world of healthcare that the findings of research with one group of people should be applicable to other settings and hence the word generalisability has higher status. This means that readers and funders can go beyond the knowledge acquired by a small piece of research. Funding bodies, in particular, expect lawlike generalities which are 'true' in different situations. Stoddard (2004) uses the term (from Kleinman, 1996) 'the folk notion of science', which gives a more abstract and simple portrait of the social world which is a characteristic of quantitative research. Funding bodies and sometimes ethics committees still believe that the knowledge gained through this type of research is more valuable than small-scale studies whose results are not generalisable. Stoddard, however, rejects this belief and explains that small-scale, qualitative research has a different kind of generalisability, and does not merely provide insight or illumination of a problem. He adopts a model of generalisability which focuses on social processes and activities. Qualitative research is more concerned with social processes rather than unchanging social structures. This Stoddard calls 'processual generalisability': it shows that social processes are generalisable beyond the specific setting to a variety of other situations. For narrative inquiry this is of particular importance as each individual tells a unique story – within a social and cultural framework, of course – and the researcher is not necessarily looking for patterns.

Example of processual generalisability
When patients tell their stories, researchers often find that there is a process of 'negotiation' with health professionals or 'struggle' with illness or an 'attempt to regain normality'. These concepts are social or psychological processes through which people pass. The research describes and illuminates these processes. The insight gained provides knowledge that can be transferred to other settings and situations and hence is generalisable, though the immediate results of the study may not be.

Olson (2001) specifically speaks of 'naturalistic generalisation' in nursing research where the unique and specific experience is important. In this type of inquiry, readers of the study have the feeling that they are present when the events and activities that have occurred are told because the researcher closely follows the experiences of the participants. Also, in reference to qualitative research in nursing, Johnson (1996) reframes the concept of generalisability by pointing to Morse and Sandelowski who, in their many writings, discuss the concept of 'theory generalisation'. However, the idea of theory generalisation is more relevant to grounded theory where the emerging theory can be applied to different groups and different contexts.

Within the idea of processual or theoretical generalisability, cases of narrative that differ greatly from other stories can also be accommodated. Although the focus is on the unique and individual stories of the person, the findings teased from these stories can be applied to a variety of settings or conditions and produce knowledge. Conventional notions of generalisation focus on verification rather than insight into unique stories that make sense to participant, researcher and reader whereas it is a more subtle concept in narrative inquiry.

The final account has to have a sense of verisimilitude; that is, when listeners hear the narrative, it should appear to be truthful. It must also have transparency in the research process, and the audit trail is a significant way to show this; all the strategies and procedures employed need to be described in sufficient detail. Coherence and contextuality are also important. Most significantly, however, the narrative should represent the meaning and reality of the participants.

The discussion of truth, in any case, is problematic. There is the question not only of the truthfulness of narrators but also the suggestion that they report only that of which they are aware. As Churchill (2000: 45) states: 'subjects can only report the "contents" of their awareness'. He refers in particular to phenomenological research in his discussion of 'narrative validity'. We have to simplify his argument, but in essence he criticises the way in which researchers discuss the 'validity' of verbal accounts. He suggests that psychologists in particular focus on the operations or mechanisms of experience rather than its understanding. Phenomenologists, he says, are not so much interested in the accuracy of self-reports but in the meanings of experience. Narratives reveal meanings and intentions. Whether self-reports are true or false, researchers suspend belief in their 'truth' to analyse the meanings inherent in them. Churchill gives a number of examples of this in phenomenology. One might advise, however, that all serious narrative researchers focus on meanings and intentions of the participants in the inquiry, even though they might not follow the processes of phenomenology.

Silverman (2005) warns about 'anecdotalism' in all forms of qualitative research. He maintains that this exists 'where research reports appear to tell entertaining stories or anecdotes but fail to convince the reader of their scientific credibility' (p. 377). The danger of this journalistic presentation increases in narrative inquiry, as it is based on stories. It is important that researchers don't just present some dramatic and interesting elements from the participants' narrative but need to demonstrate also that the findings which are generated from the stories have typicality and are representative of both the content and the meanings which participants attribute to their experience. They should also show how they analysed the narratives and arrived at their conclusions from the collected data.

It is important to remember, however, that, regardless of belief in the stories of the participants and confidence of researchers' own 'accurate' interpretation of them, researchers demonstrate that they are critical in their own thinking. A dose of healthy scepticism and doubt will send them back to their data to reflect on them and not merely take them at their face value. A further exploration of 'deviant' or negative cases is useful too; the researcher needs to be open to stories that contrast with the general tenor of the findings and account for these competing stories. In narrative inquiry, unfortunately, there are few ways to triangulate within method – for instance using observation and interviews – as there is no observation, nor are there any other forms of data collection apart from the participants' stories in whatever form they are told.

Summary

Researchers use a variety of terms to discuss the quality of their studies. In narrative research, trustworthiness and authenticity seem very appropriate. These mean that the researcher remains faithful to the meaning and experience of the participants as told in their stories, although the researcher transforms and/or interprets them. The trustworthiness and authenticity are established through a number of procedures and strategies such as the development of an audit trail and through being reflexive. The researcher must attempt to be context sensitive.

11 Problems and Critical Issues

Qualitative research, and in particular narrative inquiry, has long been seen as a balance and complement to positivist types of inquiry. Different approaches, of course, answer different types of questions. Like any other type of research, narrative inquiry contains problematic issues. Blumenreich (2004: 77) suggests that 'the method of narrative inquiry which creates the tale of an autonomous individual capable of negotiating the world in a unique way' might also generate problems like every other type of inquiry. She claims that early narrative research tended to contain a mass of raw data and the attempt by researchers to suppress their own voices and interpretation for fear of drowning the storytellers' perspectives. This, of course, neglects the fact that researchers ultimately construct the final narrative in spite of their intentions to present the voice of the participants. Blumenreich advocates that the researcher give the 'flavour' of the participants' experience and help the reader acquire sensitivity and awareness in order to capture the experiences of the participants. One could go further: not just the 'flavour' of the encounters with people in the specific context of the research is important but also the authenticity of presentation by researchers. As Todres and Galvin (2005: 2) state: 'The transferability of insights thus forgoes immediate empirical generalization but gains the human authenticity of someone living their life.'

Critical comments on narrative research often suggest that this approach is journalistic or relies on anecdotal information; so-called evidence-based research – that is, quantitative research which relies on numerical representation, measures relationships between variables and quantifies – always seems to be given privileged high status (here we must stress again that we strongly believe that this type of research is necessary to explore particular research problems, but not all questions can be answered through it). The critique of narrative inquiry is focused on the premise that it is not 'evidence based' or scientific. However, Morse (2005, 2006) presents the argument that qualitative research too is evidence based. Its data, however, are different and collected in specific contexts, relying on the thoughts and feelings of the participants. It is sometimes forgotten that people act on their perceptions and feelings, and their behaviour is rooted in these; the

Thomas theorem (Thomas and Thomas, 1928: 572) is still valid: 'If men [*sic*] define situations as real, they are real in their consequences.' People's perspectives therefore are important for nurses whether individuals' accounts are based on ostensibly 'objective' fact or not.

Also, narrative research is often carried out with a small sample of individuals, settings and situations and hence is not seen as generalisable or even transferable (see Chapter 10). Its critics sometimes seem to lack awareness that specific critical incidents and conditions as well as unique individuals are significant sources of information and are as important as patterns or generalisable ideas.

The researcher's problems

Researchers who carry out narrative research take great care that the 'voice' of the participants can be heard, and stress that these are not 'objects' but thinking human beings who present and create ideas and do not merely respond to the actions and questions of others. Nevertheless, these researchers too might objectify the participants by exploiting them. Participants are only too pleased to oblige and tell their stories because they want to help the researcher and wish to be heard. All human beings – in particular those who are ill and vulnerable – see telling their stories as an important part of their lives, hence every researcher has a responsibility to be as faithful as possible to the participants' thoughts and ideas without losing his or her own analytic stance towards these stories. Denzin (1989) distinguishes between first and second order concepts. First order concepts are the constructions developed by research participants while second order concepts are the scientific constructions that the researchers impose on the data and through which they uncover the participants' meanings. Researchers always need to base their own concepts on the constructs of the participants. This also presents narrative researchers and the reader of their accounts with complex issues. Experience is interpreted by the participants, and a second layer of interpretation, or at least a level of abstraction, is added by the researcher.

Researchers claim that stories generate rich data and allow insight into the participants' meanings which would improve clinical practice. This might be so. Sometimes they might even generate a simple understanding of complex situations. This needs evidence from the field. Initially practice might be made more difficult as researchers work with new and unforeseen knowledge derived directly from participants' stories. Even if the stories are not true, the participants' actions are based on their beliefs in the truth of their stories, and this may well assist in the healing or treatment processes. However, people also conform in their stories to cultural expectations; these might not only inform but could also distort some of the ideas presented, regardless of whether they come from patients or health professionals.

The position of the storytellers also influences the way they perceive the 'truth'. For instance, power and culture – or subculture – are linked in narratives. Patient stories may be 'counter narratives' to those of professionals, in which the former justify their actions and beliefs which may be in conflict with, or at least different from, those in control or members of perceived elite groups such as health professionals and specifically doctors. This is powerfully shown by Garro (2000) in the context of non-European culture. She explains that different explanatory models exist for doctors and patients in her study of diabetes in a Canadian community. Nevertheless, different ways of viewing and interpreting exist in any social and nursing setting. While professionals often see disease as being outside the wider social and cultural context, patients see their condition in the context of their 'lived body', their interaction with significant others, but both groups are affected by motives and expectations. Another problem can be added: it is not possible to fix the meanings given to experience by participants once and for all time; they are constantly changing as are motives and expectations.

The researchers' claims also have to be considered with their own agenda and background in mind; their subjectivity has to be taken into account. It may well be a resource in collecting and analysing information or 'having a feel' for the situation and the context, but it could also be a hindrance as it might be rooted in under-researched assumptions based on anecdotal evidence and impressions. The impressionist element of the researcher's narrative might make readers feel that they are given a portrait not based on 'real life'. Therefore the researcher has to be cautious not to add ideas based on assumptions but to analyse the data thoroughly and rely on them for meaning as well as to demonstrate an audit trail.

After all, there is a fine line between factual and fictional use of the data. The danger is most obvious when researchers use raw data in the form of quotations from participants and merely expand on these rather than going through a process of analysis (but see also some of Frank's comments later). New researchers, in particular, often make this mistake. The readers of the researcher's account understand the narrative in context – the context in which the data are collected, analysed and transformed through interpretation – and also by knowing the researcher's background and standpoint. Churchill (2000) stresses the importance of analysis. He echoes the concern of others (see Chapter 10) that stories may contain errors – particularly that of self-deception. However, he also states that researchers do not take self-reports at 'face value' but, as said before, interpret and transform the data in the process of analysis. The examples he gives are derived from phenomenology, but other narrative researchers share similar concerns, and, as Churchill (p. 47) says, shifts in participants' reports often uncover 'something fundamental about the experience'. The researcher can ask multiple questions of the data during analysis and is able to reflect on them. Participants do not merely offer descriptions of what happened to them, what they did and how they were treated, they also make meaning of their experiences and find explanations; they tell stories which include cause and effect, temporality and characters – all part of emplotment. The researcher must account for and capture this and 'fill the gaps'. On the other hand, the audience interprets the narratives through intersubjectivity as listeners understand the account of the researcher and the stories of participants on the basis of shared meanings as human beings and as members of a similar, or even common, culture to that of the researcher and the participants.

Another problem, which all qualitative researchers have in common, is the selection process the researchers undertake. They choose very specific elements from the participant stories that have relevance or are related to their own agenda and leave out much that they believe to be unrelated to the direction in which they are proceeding. To avoid this, they have to expose contrary occurrences or deviant cases, uncovering the possibilities for alternative or even competing interpretation and explanation. However, they cannot prevent some form of selection of that which they deem appropriate and useful for their final narrative.

Analysis and social structure

Atkinson (1997) and Atkinson and Silverman (1997), in two groundbreaking articles, engaged in a debate about personal narratives and biographical research. Much of this is still relevant for researchers who use narrative inquiry. Atkinson and Silverman observe the preoccupation of qualitative researchers with personal narratives and criticise the claims that these are a privileged form of access to individual experiences, 'the elevation of the experiential as the authentic' (p. 3). They also believe that researchers often are uncritical and develop an 'unexamined model of the social actor'. Atkinson in particular is sceptical about some of authors of this type of research, notably Kleinman, Mishler and Frank, deploring the lack of 'context, social action and interaction' (Atkinson, 1997: 339). He criticises the absence of culture and social structure, 'the social order', particularly in the work of Arthur Frank which he feels is devoid of 'serious social analysis' and who gives more significance to some types of narrative than to others. For instance, he accuses Frank of privileging autobiographical work and lay narratives over those of professionals. Atkinson's argument is complex, and we can only summarise some of it. Bury (2001) adds his own arguments and warning on narrative research. Within the debate on narratives and identity, he suggests that the experiences of individuals who suffer pain and illness are sometimes described in sentimental terms by themselves and researchers. The latter might reproduce their stories uncritically or without reflection. The context of their lives and their relationships in which the experiences are located are often forgotten by an overemphasis on 'personal stories'. The critics seem to focus on the romanticism and, possibly, the self-indulgence of self-revelation.

Frank (2000) responds to this criticism of his and others' work. Although he welcomes Atkinson's critique, he points out that storytellers are not always aware of the structures which are inherent in their stories, while the researcher does explicate these. The structures are not important in Frank's view because narrative research focuses on that which is significant for storytellers. As far as social context is concerned, it is involved in the relationship of the storyteller to the listeners and readers of the stories, and reaffirms 'who they are with respect to each other' (2000: 354), involving relationships and community. He claims the 'recuperative role' of storytelling and emphasises that stories are more than data for analysis, and that narrative research should focus on the participants rather than the researcher. The research is imbued with values and ethical acts, and Frank sees this as an asset rather than accepting it as a criticism. He also rejects Atkinson's claim that advocacy in narrative research is not legitimate, maintaining that the therapeutic effect on the storyteller, and the 'moral imagination that allows listening without the imposition of analytic categories', are important for the researcher. The work is specifically not about medical or professional tales but focuses on ill persons' stories which are often silenced by those of professionals. The complexity of these arguments suggests that researchers become acquainted with the debate by reading these articles.

Interpretation and meaning

The issue of the hidden, 'unsayable' and 'invisible' can also be a problem for the researcher. Rogers et al. (1999) suggest that researchers should attempt to see, hear and interpret more than that which they can directly capture which cannot always be expressed in words. Qualitative researchers are often warned by well known writers not to invent ideas and firmly ground them in the data, but the opposite might also apply: they do not always grasp the unsaid or invisible; this, Rogers and her colleagues suggest, can add something valuable to the researcher's own narrative. Narrative inquiry is uniquely placed to make the unsaid heard or the invisible visible. When the story is read from transcription, it is merely text to be analysed, but when it is initially heard, it consists of spoken words and has immediacy. Long silences, gestures and facial features may express emotion or ambiguity in the participant. The dynamic of interaction may be lost in the written story – the transcript; feelings revealed through interaction relationships are an integral part of the story. The researcher should remember emotions which are significant elements in experience and influence human thought and behaviour, though they are often neglected in research. No health researcher can afford to miss these. Through their own account of the participant stories, they might make them visible. This, after all, is one of the most important issues in narrative inquiry.

To give a fair account of participants' stories is in itself problematic. Nelson and McGillion (2004: 633) suggest that participants use their experience selectively in stories, and advise listeners not to assume that 'there exists any "pure space" from which voices speak'. Participants choose elements not only from their experience or knowledge that they think appropriate and 'revealable' to the research situation but also from a range of styles available to them. This means that the stories are rarely 'mere' descriptions of an experience. Indeed Nelson and McGillion claim that participants build an 'acceptable self' in stories. The story told is thus a preferred version from a range of possibilities. They might tend to narrate what they feel is acceptable – to themselves and others – in the research situation, the story which puts them in a good light, and, most of all, which holds the interest of the listener. From our own reading we find that dramatic and interesting stories are preferable to researchers but the ordinary might be just as important.

The truth of stories

One of the problems of all narrative and interviewing research is that of truth (see Chapter 10). Atkinson et al. (2003) have discussed this in relation to earlier debates. How does the researcher know that the participant is telling the truth? Is the 'objective' truth important? Is there a single 'absolute truth'? The truth, these authors maintain, is 'unknowable', but they demand examination of this concept, and the debate is long and complex. However, Atkinson et al. claim that there is no need to either believe or reject the accounts of participants as long as a proper analytic stance towards them is adopted. It is important, however, to examine 'the vocabulary of motive', a term used by Mills (1940) to signify that which drives the participant to tell the story in a particular way.

Of course, the researcher is interested not only in facts or the 'truth' of the participants' stories but also in their motivation. Emotional and factual/rational description may both be part of the story. The issues or problems illustrated are not dependent, however, on the factual accuracy of the story (Phillips, 1997). Of course, the better the stories fit into the cultural and social framework of the listener, the more credible they become. Indeed, Spence (1982) speaks of 'historical truth and narrative truth', the former being what in fact happened, the latter about the decision people make to capture their experience as a whole. Narrative truth can convince the reader of the story told. Internal contradictions or inconsistencies in the participants' stories may, however, become an issue for exploration and discussion.

Stories and memory

Linked to the problem of truth telling is the issue of memory. This in turn is connected with a multiplicity of concepts and terms such as recall, recollection and review, for instance, all with different but similar meanings. (For the purpose of this debate these are not of major importance. For a longer discussion see Roberts, 2002: 134–150.) Memory is linked to the perception of self as well as to the social context. When individuals review the past, they remember what it meant for them, how it fits into their self-concept and the wider process of their lives. Memory is selective, and different aspects of it might even compete with each other, before the one is chosen that is deemed most appropriate at the time. The link to the present and future is unmistakable. The importance of temporality and social construction emerges again. It should also be remembered that memory can change or be reorganised according to circumstances. This is not fiction but the way in which individuals perceive situations retrospectively. The researcher, although aware of all these issues, will obtain the perspectives and perceptions of the participants about their situation and experience as they remember them at the time when the stories are collected.

Self-critique and critique by others

Narrative researchers often have immense enthusiasm and are convinced of the value of this type of research. This means, just occasionally, that they are not self-critical or reflective enough about their work or about narrative inquiry itself which has its problems just as does every other type of research. The approach may end up as a mere retelling of stories and lack analysis and insight. It needs robustness and hard work, although sensitivity and empathy with the participants are at its heart.

As said before, narrative research places much emphasis on the reader of the text to do the work, which could be seen to be a problem; however, most postmodernists see this as part of the underpinning philosophy of narrative inquiry in that multiple readings of texts can co-exist. One of the concerns from more traditional research quarters is that this assumes a relativistic stance.

With the increased need for reflexivity and the intensity of both the relationship and the data, narrative research is labour intensive, particularly around emotional labour. It actually requires more commitment of self to the process, which of course is not always desired. From a traditional point of view narrative research is viewed as primitive and savage, and underdeveloped, which is why it lacks credibility with the traditionalists, but of course their own research is created by and through narrative too; this is the only way it can tell itself.

Summary

Critics point out that narrative inquiry does not have a more privileged status than other types of research. The critique of narrative research also focuses on the potential lack of 'truth' by the participants, but we have pointed to the importance of their perceptions which, for them, are 'truths'. Narrative researchers try to demonstrate that there is no absolute 'truth' in any case.

Like any type of research, narrative inquiry has also generated critique and criticism, not least because it is seen as non-scientific by traditionalists.

Practical Considerations

12 Writing for Publication and Other Ways of Disseminating Narrative Research

Silverman (2005) suggests that dissemination is part of the aftermath of carrying out research and a necessary step. There are several ways of disseminating research:

(1) Publishing articles in reputable and, if possible, peer reviewed journals.
(2) Writing a monograph or chapter in a book.
(3) Presenting papers at conferences.
(4) Sharing information in the workplace.
(5) Using performance based methods such as theatre and role play or interactive websites.

There is no point in researching and writing if the findings of the research do not reach the diverse audiences and readership to which they can be useful. Publishing narrative research does not differ much from publishing other types of inquiry. After all, narrative inquiry in nursing is not undertaken as 'blue skies' research but has the purpose of assisting nurses to carry out their professional tasks. It is, however, a little more difficult – though not impossible – to publish qualitative research, and specifically narrative studies, in respected and reputable academic journals. The quantitative paradigm still predominates, particularly in medical and other healthcare journals, although good qualitative studies are now more prevalent in nursing and healthcare journals than ten or twenty years ago. Medical journals only started publishing qualitative articles more frequently in the last decade.

Performances in theatre, film and role play can often be effective in presenting narrative research (Jones, 2005a) in a more immediate way. In our own university we attended a seminar which showed the outcome of research in a piece of theatre in which the 'actors' – mostly experienced health professionals – acted out the story of a group of people who were interacting with a dying patient. Their thoughts, problems and sadness were demonstrated in a short play. Participants in the role play felt that this might have been a better way of depicting the situation than talking about it in a presentation at a conference or a written article. This way of presenting narrative research is becoming more common. Keen and Todres (2006: 13) give a list of types of dissemination for qualitative research which include, among others, research-based drama, dance, workshops, film and poetic texts as well as websites.

Websites might be a particularly useful and appropriate way of dissemination. The DIPEx website (www.DIPEx.org), for instance, is a resource where patients, carers and others can share the experiences and stories of people who have an illness or a health problem. Researchers might produce a website in a similar way to disseminate the findings of their research.

There are of course, a number of reasons for publication and other forms of dissemination:

(1) *The advance in knowledge.* Even a small piece of narrative research will add to the stock of knowledge and information in the specific field of study. Most well known writers, including Strauss and Corbin (1998), suggest that knowledge cannot be increased or accumulated if it is kept private and not made public. Even if other articles or books have been written in the area of research, a phenomenon needs to be illuminated from many angles for it to become clear and understandable in depth. Dissemination also challenges established beliefs – an important point – and starts a debate about a particular issue which helps in the progression of knowledge (Holloway and Walker, 2000). The debate itself might show development in the field of study, and this is important.

(2) *Raising awareness about people's conditions and their perspectives.* Patient stories and researcher narratives assist health professionals to learn about the feelings and thoughts of their clients and hence to learn how to respond.

(3) *The enhancement of the researcher's reputation and profile through publication.* Through this they advance their career and increase their standing and reputation in the organisation in which they work. Sharing newly acquired knowledge and thoughts about it is a process that is useful for the readership of the publication and enjoyable for the researcher. Researchers gain credibility in their discipline or make a name for themselves through an unusual approach to a subject area. Publication and presentation at conferences also help new researchers to gain confidence.

(4) *Claiming ownership.* Occasionally others in the field carry out similar research. We know of cases where good ideas of one researcher have been used by others before the researcher had the chance to publish them as his or her own ideas. Publication lays claim to owning the ideas put forward, if they are new, or if an unusual route and approach have been followed.

(5) *Dissemination raises the profile of the institution.* To gain research funds, the reputation of universities needs to be high. The higher the discipline rates in the Research Assessment Exercise, the better the funding from a variety of sources.

Albarran and Scholes (2005) claim that academics often judge colleagues by their profile in research and publications. Practitioners in clinical practice too feel the need to disseminate their work. Publications contribute to information about the problem of the theory–practice gap and how it can be solved, as well as increasing knowledge about theory and practice development.

Dissemination may occur through articles in journals (including electronic sites), books, posters and various ways of presenting at conferences and meetings.

Writing an article for the appropriate journal

It is necessary to look at a number of journals to choose one whose aim, content and layout are appropriate for the study. To find the right journal in which to publish, writers have to ask themselves the following questions:

- What aspects of my research should be published?
- Which readership should I address?

Researchers have to be mindful of the readership (or audience) of their dissemination strategy. Academic peers or clinical practitioners need somewhat different ways of addressing their audience. Researchers often publish solely for their peers – usually in academic journals for reasons of reputation, career enhancement and the Research Assessment Exercise. If the research is important for clinical practice, it needs to reach a wider readership of professionals who work in the field. This does not mean watering down the research to make it 'simple' for this group of people, but the article must be written in clear and understandable language for those who have not been initiated into the esoteric and theoretical terminology of academe.

The contents of the article

Researchers have to consider the 'so what' factor first, namely whether the written article is worth publishing and the content is significant and interesting for their peers. In an academic journal the contribution must be at a level comparable to that of other publications in the same journal and achieve an academic standard. The most common submissions contain a description of the methodology and strategies, ethical issues, and, most importantly, the findings and discussion of these in summary form and in a conventional way. Most academic journal editors favour this type of presentation although they do value originality of presentation too (for instance the journals *Qualitative Inquiry* and *Narrative Inquiry*, though these are not specifically for nurses). The methods section commonly includes the strategies the researcher adopted: the setting, the sample, the strategies of data collection and analysis and a rationale for the approach. The findings and discussion sections in an article on narrative research might be either integrated or discussed separately. There is not usually a long literature review as the dialogue with the literature occurs in the discussion of particular themes that emerge. (More detail on the use of literature can be found in Chapters 6 and 9.) Journals have guidelines for submission and publication either in the early pages or at the end. Karen Dahlberg (2006) discusses the dilemma of presentation and publication of qualitative research. She claims that the publication of findings is integral to the research and indeed affects it. Because of the limitations of many journals on word numbers (and other issues of course), it is more difficult to publish this type of research. Qualitative inquiry, and in particular narrative analysis, need space because of methodological issues – such as the need for more detailed description of the methodology and audit trail. We would add that the journal should not shape the form in which the article is being written: the research itself should determine the journals in which researchers publish.

Many researchers carry out 'salami slicing' with their study. They might publish a discussion of a particular ethical or methodological problem that occurred in the research and present its solution. Sometimes they demonstrate how a theory or theories grounded in the data illustrate the topic in a new and original way. An interesting and novel illumination of the literature relating to the topic is another favoured way of shaping an article. Researchers also may give a detailed account of a specific theme that emerged from people's narratives. The 'slices', however, must have substance and contribute to the knowledge on narrative research and not repeat the ideas from the research that have already been published.

The presentation of narrative research may be difficult. The researcher must give an audit trail and a more detailed description of methodology and findings which might make it longer than articles based on quantitative forms of inquiry. It is more appropriate, therefore, to use journals that specifically publish qualitative research such as *Qualitative Health Research*, *Narrative Research*, *Qualitative Research*, *Narrative Inquiry* or the electronic *International Journal of Qualitative*

Methods. There are others, particularly in education and sociology. However, the researcher has to consider a wider audience. How can we as qualitative researchers ever gain recognition of the value of our studies, if we only present their results to like-minded peers? Often narrative research challenges firmly held beliefs and assumptions that are held about an area of interest.

The length of articles also differs between journals; some publish up to 6000 words, others accept shorter pieces, and others put sections on the web and publish the main summary of the research. It is important to be crisp and succinct, even in accounts of narrative research. The publication gains more respect from peers if there are mainly primary references and not references from secondary sources.

Style of writing

Narrative research publications have their own inimical style as we have mentioned before. The writer has to be true to the character of the narrators' stories as well as to his or her own way of writing. The type of journal and the wishes of publishers too have to be taken into account. Christine Webb (1992, 2002) has waged a campaign about style in journal writing. She has always advocated the use of the first person in writing research articles – singular or plural as appropriate – particularly keeping in mind that authors should acknowledge their responsibility and be accountable for their actions. Rather than saying 'data were collected', the author might write 'I collected data'. It is pretentious to write about oneself as 'the author' or 'the researcher'. Use of the passive tense or stilted writing makes the article less lively and dynamic. This applies particularly to narrative research, where writers need an interesting story and to make the research readable. Gilgun too (2005: 258) advises researchers to take personal responsibility for their writing. She quotes Haraway (1988) who warned writers not to use the 'god trick' by staying anonymous and not using the first person voice. The use of the active voice also enlivens the writing unlike the presentation of a passive disembodied perspective.

A clear layout and organisation can persuade reviewers that the researcher has a good understanding of his or her own research and has followed a logical process. A good title and an interesting abstract demonstrate to reviewer and reader that the article has merit. Davis and Shadle (2000) regret that academic writing is so often lifeless and routine. They claim that researchers often provide standardised, unoriginal articles which show detachment and certainty rather than 'a new valuation of uncertainty, passionate exploration and mystery' (p. 418). We believe that this is particularly important when writing narrative research articles which, after all, are designed to draw the reader into the narrative and experience of participants so that the reader can evaluate them and learn from the findings. Davis and Shadle suggest writing alternative possibilities, such as argumentative or personal research papers, while advising researchers to adhere to academic standards and evidence. To write in alternative ways, of course, the writer has to know the conventions of 'ordinary' social science articles and presentations. The research argument sets out a thesis and arguments for and against it. In a way the debate is a conversation of researchers with themselves and also with the related literature, giving both interpretations and alternative perspectives on the phenomenon and finishing with a convincing explanation for the varying interpretations and their own perception of the findings.

Peer review of articles

Articles are sent for review to other researchers who will read 'blind', that is, they won't know the name or the affiliation of the writer, nor will the writer find out who has reviewed the work. Editors attempt to find reviewers who know the topic and/or the methodology – although this is not always so, particularly now that academics are so busy and don't have the time to review many articles during their academic year. Reviewers send detailed comments to the editor of the journal who passes them on to the writer. In the past, professional journals did not go through the same rigorous review process as academic publications do, but they are now scrutinised carefully as their editors too are very keen to receive high quality articles and most are reviewed. Professional journals generally have a wider readership in nursing.

When an article is returned for revision, writers usually look at each of the comments in turn and try to address them one by one. The editor expects either a change or an explanation in answer to the query, and he or she decides whether the article can be published in the revised form or should be rejected. Some articles are submitted to the journal several times. Usually an article improves after researchers follow some of the advice of the referees. Occasionally, however, writers – ourselves included – feel that reviewers have not understood the topic, or, more likely, do not know the qualitative research approach very well. Often, instead of entering an argument, researchers follow the guidance of reviewers as they wish to be published. Frey (2003) argues that there is danger inherent in this: authors sometimes intellectually prostitute themselves by following the advice of referees. Nevertheless, most researchers realise that they can always learn from others and gain a fresh viewpoint on their study. Following at least some of the advice may well enhance the article (or book).

In general the reviewers recommend to the editor of the journal one of several actions, outright rejection of the article, immediate acceptance, or revision (either major or minor). Journal editors do not usually accept articles that have also been submitted elsewhere. However, a rejected article sometimes finds favour in another, less demanding journal, or in one that takes a different perspective on the same topic, is more in tune with the aim of the research or is more suitable and appropriate for the area of study. If rejected, the author can take into account the suggestions of the reviewers and send it to a different, perhaps more appropriate journal. It is advisable, if at all possible, to make the suggested amendments to the article. Usually the article will eventually be accepted, often after the first revision. It is rare for an article to be accepted without even minor amendments. If authors feel that something has been misunderstood or that the comments are based on a different approach (and this does sometimes happen in qualitative research articles), they can respond to the review, but these tactics should be adopted only in exceptional circumstances. It is better to give in gracefully and make amendments while still staying honest and true to the original content and approach. In their initial stages of attempting to publish, writers might be very hurt to be criticised and even rejected when so much work has gone into an article. Criticism, however, tends to make us think about what we have written. Most researchers become used to having articles rejected at some stage of their career. There is rarely an author whose work has never been rejected.

The technical process of writing and publishing an article

Newell (2000: 94) gives good advice on starting a piece of writing for a journal, namely 'to calibrate the task and then work on each element of it'. This means writing a structure and filling in the gaps between – though they might not be the headings of the article, nor does this have to be done sequentially at the planning stage. The author needs to decide how much to write under each of these headings. A journal article has more chance of being published if its grammar and spelling are correct. Journal editors get irritated by avoidable mistakes though they do not necessarily reject the article. All research articles need to be explicit about the aim, the methodology and procedures, the topic area and findings of the research, and they must have a conclusion. Even readers who have been trained in quantitative methods should be able to understand an article in which the writer uses a narrative approach.

The authors also have to point out the gaps in the literature which they want to fill. For professional journals and clinical readership it is essential to include implications for practice, although many academic reviewers also welcome this.

The problems of publishing narrative research

There are particular problems involved in publishing all qualitative research. In the past, editors were not used to qualitative research in general and narrative inquiry in particular, and sometimes they judged it from the standpoint of the quantitative paradigm. This has changed recently, and many journal editors – except perhaps those of the most 'scientific' medical ones – are quite happy to publish qualitative research as long as they think it is rigorous and has high quality. As said before, some edit journals that aim to publish qualitative research.

However, there is the problem of quality in narrative research. If publishers and peers disagree with the concept of validity in qualitative research (or equivalent concepts specific for this type of inquiry), they might see narrative health research as less 'generalisable' than other types of approach. Most stakeholders and health professionals believe that, to be useful, research results have to be applicable to a variety, indeed a large number, of settings and similar situations. Narrative research is situation-specific and context-bound to a potentially small number of situations and contexts, and the researcher has to make explicit the importance of the study to other areas and similar situations (see the chapter on trustworthiness) otherwise it might not be seen as 'valid' or useful. Even the nature of sampling in narrative inquiry works against the narrative researcher in the quantitative world.

Publishing a book

Researchers often decide to publish a book on their research, especially if the topic is interesting and important for professional or academic peers or if it deals with unexplored but significant areas of nursing. Writing a book is now much easier than in earlier times because publishers are keen to expand their portfolio and their markets. Publishers do wish to enhance their reputation with their published book, but they also want to know whether the book will sell and increase their profits; therefore the market to which they sell will have to be reasonably large. However great a book, if the title and topic are obscure and the potential readership is small, a publisher will be reluctant to publish. Researchers who wish to publish their PhD in particular will find it difficult to publish their research in a monograph although occasionally it may happen (such as the text on the emotional labour of nursing by Pam Smith (1992) or on learning and working by Kath Melia (1987) who both used their PhD research and expanded on it for their now very well known books). All publishers have proposal sheets in which they attempt to get detailed information from writers about the content, level, readership and market of the proposed text as well as about similar competitive books.

The time from conception to the final publication of a book varies and normally depends on the speed and writing skill of the author as well as on the timetable of the publisher. Commissioning editors make the rounds of universities and might approach academics, but the latter might write to or phone a publisher to discuss the publication of a book. Obviously it is important to seek a reputable firm whose editors commission books in the same discipline or area of study as that of the writer. It is in the interest of both publisher and writer to get the book out reasonably quickly for a variety of reasons, but publication is a lengthy process which includes copy editing, proofreading and indexing, some of which is undertaken by the author. We have been lucky with our publishers and their flexibility, but there are some who are either very slow in preparing the final copy, or they push the author relentlessly to hand in the book. In both clinical and academic circles, writers have full-time jobs and sometimes find it difficult to complete on time.

A book might be valued by its readership and enhance the reputation of the organisation in which the author works, but it does not seem to have the same impact as an article in a published journey for the Research Assessment Exercise and is sometimes rated lower by academic peers because it does not have the same critical review as do journal articles. However, the same writing rules about spelling, grammar and appropriateness for the readership apply to books as to journal articles, except that the latter are really a summary of what the author wants to say to readers while a book makes it explicit.

Often researchers contribute to chapters in an edited book which deals with the topic area of the study; an example is the book by Hurwitz et al. (2004) on narrative research in health and illness.

Ethical issues in dissemination

It is obvious that researchers should not present other people's intellectual property or take credit for their work. Most researchers act ethically towards their research participants as well as towards their peers. If anything is paraphrased, the source of the idea must be cited and verbatim statements need quotation marks and reference to author and page number. Plagiarism is mentioned in many chapters and books on publication, but we feel that we are already 'preaching to the converted'. Lately emphasis has also been placed on self-plagiarism: even one's own ideas previously published should be referenced. There is now also controversy about sequential work on the development and phases of a research project, but we feel that this is legitimate as long as different issues are discussed in these articles. After all, most authors cannot squeeze all important issues into a single article because significant issues have to be explicated and discussed rather than merely summarised. Journal editors generally want articles that are not submitted elsewhere at the same time. For tables or larger amounts of material from other authors which the writer wishes to use, he or she has to obtain permission from the publisher or the author. Some novice authors do not know that this has to be done.

The main ethical issue is linked to the faithful presentation of the participants' ideas. Their voices must be heard in the book or article about a narrative research endeavour. Their rights should be protected. Anonymity and confidentiality are of paramount importance, and the author's ethical integrity is essential.

We have added a short checklist for articles and book chapters which are based on narrative research (some of these criteria also have importance for books, book chapters or oral presentations):

- Is the article true to the character of narrative inquiry?
- Does the article have the appropriate level for the journal and the intended readership?
- Are the material and topic of importance for nurses?
- Does the researcher explore a novel, interesting and important topic area?
- Does the article explicate and cover ethical issues in the research?
- Does the article have a theoretical framework (for academic journals)?
- Will the research illuminate a clinical problem (particularly for professional journals)?
- Is the writing clear and unambiguous?
- Does the author contribute to the scholarly discussion of the topic?

Giving oral presentations at conferences or meetings

Oral presentations of papers are significantly different from articles, although they are often preliminary to publication of articles in journals. These differences are linked to the context and audience (rather than readership). Though articles too are based on interpersonal interaction to an extent, this interaction is neither as simultaneous nor as immediate as that in presentations at conferences (Rowley-Jolivet and Carter-Thomas, 2005).

The presentation has to be honed down from the rich data elicited in the research and needs to be linked to the research topic as well as the theme of the conference. The researcher directs the presentation towards the specific audience of the paper. This means an awareness of the background of delegates in the conference, that is, their professional or academic position. A conference involving only students will be quite different from that comprising academics and PhD candidates. The audience might also include professionals from clinical settings who need a different focus. The most difficult presentation is the one aimed at a mixed audience involving people with different perspectives and ideologies.

Practical issues in presentations

There are some practical issues about presenting conference papers. Usually the presentation of these papers lasts between 30 and 40 minutes including questions from the audience. The initial abstract of course is a response to the 'call for papers' from the conference organisers and should follow their guidelines and specific format. This abstract is of importance as acceptance for the conference presentation depends on it.

As in articles, the researcher needs a clear aim and structure for the paper and it is best to state these in the beginning (for instance: The aim of this presentation is . . . I intend to cover the following points . . .). Often researchers use overheads or PowerPoint, mainly to remind themselves and the audience of the key issues of the presentation. However, this is not necessary as long as the paper is clear and unambiguous, both in ideas and presentation (this includes producing audible and well paced sentences while using eye contact with the people in the room). It is useful to give handouts with a summary including the main points.

Many presentations go over the allotted time span; this is discourteous to other presenters whose session will be shortened as a result. It also troubles conference administrators as they have to take breaks and meals into account.

It is useful to anticipate questions, arguments and criticism that the audience might have at the end of the paper. Novice presenters may get upset at this, but, in an academic or professional environment, questions and argument are useful devices to think about the research and the questions arising from it. This enhances and develops knowledge. We have found that most of our work has improved through constructive criticism and debate.

Presenting in the workplace and to specialist groups

Many researchers work in a professional setting where few people know much about the work carried out by colleagues. Reporting on narrative research in particular can arouse the interest of peers and special groups as it is intriguing and follows a storyline. The participants themselves also value a presentation of their combined thoughts on a topic near to their lives, and the researchers can show their gratitude to them by making their voices heard.

We have found that, when writers look back at the research articles and books they have published, they gain great satisfaction from seeing their work in print. Other types of dissemination are equally useful to share the information with others. Researchers know that if the research is valid it has also been worthwhile as its findings have been disseminated and can be acted on by others as the dissemination contributes to the store of knowledge in the field.

Summary

We have discussed a number of strategies for dissemination of narrative research including articles in journals and papers, and through performative methods and workshops. The peer review process might be lengthy but usually enhances the account of the researcher. The reasons for publication and dissemination are manifold, but the most important issue is to share the knowledge acquired through narrative inquiry so that it can help in the practice or educational setting.

13 Practical Issues in Narrative Research

Narrative researchers will meet a number of practical issues and problems, especially when they are new to the process of this type of research. Some of these issues are the same or at least similar in other types of qualitative inquiry; some differ in a variety of aspects. It also requires a unique set of skills, particularly in regard to facilitating the researcher–participant relationship. Whilst many nurses are already experienced in managing relationships, they may need help to translate those skills to the research setting.

Recording and transcribing narrative data

In all qualitative research texts, writers point to the importance of recording data fully and accurately. In narrative research the stories of the participants must be grasped in their richness and flavour, in detail and nuance.

Using the tape recorder and taking notes

As researchers might only remember the main storyline and not the detail of the participants' tales, the verbal data should be tape recorded and transcribed if at all possible. We advise this in spite of the conflicting views of writers who suggest note taking only; we have found in our own studies that some elements of the participants' stories are easily forgotten or are remembered inappropriately. It is difficult to focus on the participants and their words while taking notes. Indeed tape recording is an essential step in the research process and is carried out unless the storytellers refuse permission or feel inhibited by the recorder. We have not had any refusals to record, but researchers occasionally find resistance in some participants in which case copious notes are taken – though these are better written at completion of the particular story to which they are listening. However, in some settings where tape recording is prohibited, for example in prisons, the researcher must be more sensitive to both the environment and the participants.

In narrative research video recording is rare unless the story is told in visual terms. Audio tapes are made during the storytelling process; in practical and ethical terms this means asking for permission to record, and placing the recorder near the participant so that the words can be clearly heard. The craft of narrative interviewing demands that there be a few early questions or prompts which stimulate the narrators to tell their stories. The whole process is about the stories of the participants! They soon get used to the tape recorder; indeed many claim that this is the first time that their story has been fully told and heard. Some researchers take notes throughout, but this might draw their attention away from the participants, decrease eye contact and disturb the flow of the story. It is often useful, however, to take fieldnotes too, soon after completion, in order to remember some detail of the behaviour and demeanour of the storyteller. Tapes also unveil the sound of voice and the pauses or hesitations of the participants. Patton (2002: 382) advises researchers on some important issues before, during and after the process and gives a whole page of tips for tape recording qualitative data. We have adapted these for narrative research as uninterrupted stories are of particular importance (important ethical issues are not repeated here as they are discussed in Chapter 5).

The tape recorder and tapes (60-minute tapes for better quality) should be high quality.

- The researcher needs to carry several replacement tapes for lengthy stories
- A quiet and undisturbed setting is necessary for uninterrupted talk
- The initial questions put the participants at ease and can be factual and biographical
- The few initial questions to elicit the story should focus broadly on the topic and interest of the researcher as well on as that of the participant
- If the participant becomes disturbed or uneasy, the recorder needs to be switched off
- The researcher thanks the participant
- At the end the tape is labelled with a coding number or pseudonym of the participant
- The tape is safely locked away until and again after transcription

The time for keeping the tapes differs with different institutions and guidelines. Usually they would be kept for between five and ten years unless participants object to this.

It is important to note that many people disclose significant thoughts and feelings after the tape has been turned off; these become part of the story although the researcher must make sure of ongoing permission for this. Indeed at any time when the participant reveals intimate, private and sensitive issues, the researcher will be aware of confidentiality and ask for permission to 'use' these data. Tapes are the reflection of the initial story and have to be read repeatedly, but they can never fully replace the initial oral data as researchers cannot see the face and demeanour of the participants. The descriptive and theoretical notes made after each interview should capture some of the atmosphere, the stance of participants and initial interpretations.

Transcripts of data

Transcripts are handwritten or typed passages from the tapes recorded with the participant stories (Holloway, 1997). We must stress the initial need for fact sheets which consist of facts about date, place, pseudonym and code number or letter of the participant, and any other biographical facts which might help the research process such as gender or age.

Advice on transcribing data in the form of stories varies. Many researchers transcribe their own tapes because in narrative research they wish to become truly familiar and intimate with the words of the participants. It also helps to protect anonymity and confidentiality of the individuals taking part. As the process of transcription is so long, however (four to six hours per one hour of tape), some researchers find it more productive to listen repeatedly to the tapes and ask a professional transcriber or typist to carry out the transcription. In the latter case, the person transcribing the data needs to make the same commitment as the researcher to keep confidentiality and, if recognising the voices of the participants, not to reveal their identities.

The reasons for recording and transcribing data and keeping recordings and transcripts include the following:

- To gain a full and holistic 'Gestalt' of the story
- To help the researcher's memory and accuracy
- Just as a tape can be heard many times, the transcript can be read repeatedly and analysed in detail
- In case of accusations of fraud or deception, official agencies might be able to scrutinise the integrity of the researcher

Researchers can never wholly transcribe the tapes so that all nuances of the speech are visible on paper. The transcription needs to be as accurate as possible without losing clarity.

To assist the researcher in finding specific data, we would argue for line-by-line numbering of each script and wide margins so that coding and notes can be made. A space between interviewer talk and participant story is also useful as are different fonts for researcher and participant. A transcript will show clearly whether this was a depth interview or a true narrative.

Transcribing systems do exist for conversation and discourse analysis, and could be useful, but beginners might develop their own form of notation in transcribing, for instance, *italics* for words they want to emphasise, three full stops . . . to indicate pauses, or spaced dots . . . to indicate something that has been left out. The transcriber might indicate where laughter, coughing, hesitation or distress has occurred. Accurate transcripts are important but they can never take the place of the recorded tape where every nuance of the story is audible.

The use of quotes and quotations in the final researcher narrative

Quotes in the form of excerpts from the tales of the participants are necessary evidence for the statements made by researchers (this is also discussed in Chapter 9). Writers must avoid slanting the study by an inappropriate and highly selective use of these. This can be achieved by peer review (keeping in mind confidentiality) and reflexivity. A string of quotes from all participants for each statement made is unnecessary and disturbs the flow of the study.

Direct quotations are excerpts from other sources such as the research literature or other people's comments and writings. They can lend authenticity to the research or, indeed, refute and challenge it. Usually, the writer summarises and paraphrases others' ideas and gives the source of these ideas. A direct quotation needs not only the name of the author but also the page number where it is quoted. Quotations are used when researchers might not be able to express the ideas in their own words or when they are a well known statement by an author. An example would be the quotation of the Thomas theorem, for instance, which we used elsewhere in this book.

As said before, quotes and quotations are always attributed (quotes from participants with pseudonyms, letters or numbers). The reasons for inserting the specific quotes from the stories and quotations from other sources need explanation. Too many long quotes might clutter up the write-up. Omission of words inside quotes or quotations needs indication through three dots divided by space (such as . . .). All quotes and quotations are embedded in the context of the presentation.

Evaluation of narrative research

In this section we shall summarise the characteristics of narrative research and the specific criteria by which it can be evaluated. When judging the usefulness, quality and appropriateness of narrative inquiry, its readers search for and use various ways to evaluate. Most qualitative researchers set up criteria different from those used in quantitative research, although 'criteriology' has recently been criticised by Seale (1999) and Parker (2004) in particular. Parker contends that some of the most innovative ideas in quantitative inquiry have been carried out by those who broke the rules of accepted criteria; only in this way can progress be made. Criteria, so Parker argues, should be flexible guidelines in any case, not rigid rules and conventions. Nevertheless, if narrative researchers wish to demonstrate the quality of their research to the readers of their work, whether they have quantitative or qualitative orientations, they have to develop a framework by which narrative research can be judged.

We shall discuss in summary form the essential features of the areas to be appraised and provide a checklist of the criteria for evaluation. It must, however, be noted that the quality of narrative inquiry does not depend solely on these criteria. The main judgement depends on its appropriateness, relevance, holism, credibility – and readability.

The research question or problem

The research question has to be sufficiently broad to be appropriate for, and have 'fit' with, a narrative approach. Usually the researcher wishes to examine a phenomenon, to explore the life world or centre on a specific experience and its meaning for the participant. If the intention is to develop theory, for instance, narrative inquiry is inappropriate.

The research question has close links with the aim of the research and reflects it. Most important in framing a research question, however, is that it demonstrates the contribution to nursing knowledge that it can make.

Research methodology and design

The rationale of the research will explain the choice of methodology and the way it is rooted in a particular philosophy. It is important that researchers discuss the underlying philosophy of narrative research. The background and the empirical setting are described in fair detail so that the reader gains a picture of the context.

'Embeddedness' in context

The term 'embeddedness' is used by Greenhalgh et al. (2005) to show that all narrative research is integral to its context. The researcher needs to be context intelligent and sensitive to the setting and people involved. The social situation of the research with all its complexities is spelt out in fair detail and the research engages with 'real life situations' (Fossey et al., 2002). Researchers also describe the context in which the participants live as well as their own location, so that the readers have awareness and grasp of it.

The literature

The initial literature review does not direct the study but instead demonstrates the gaps in knowledge and the place where researchers can contribute new ideas to the field. In the discussion section the literature is interwoven with the debate on specific themes or ideas, and researchers demonstrate that it confirms their own ideas or challenges them. The main literature sections are always integrated in the text rather than discussed in detail in the beginning of the study.

Sampling

Narrative sampling usually includes few participants as the uniqueness of their story, or the depth of the phenomenon embedded in it, is important rather than breadth. Researchers describe the scope and limitations of this sample and how he or she gained access to it. The term 'subject' is not appropriate as it might objectify the participants, although we have occasionally seen it used.

Data collection and analysis

The researcher describes the way in which narrative interviews have been carried out as previously explained in more detail. Narrative interviews, so-called, although they do not take the same question and in-depth answer form of other qualitative interviews, differ in that the answers are contained in longer stories and the narrators develop their response.

Ethical considerations

Among major ethical issues which should be discussed, researchers also show that the specifics of narrative ethics are taken into account, particularly in the areas of informed consent and anonymity. The need for ongoing consent is stressed.

Validity or trustworthiness

If the term 'validity' is used, the researcher clarifies that validity in narrative inquiry has a different meaning from that in quantitative research.

The explanations of trustworthiness or validity, and the steps taken for ensuring it, will be described. This section should demonstrate that an audit trail exists, that peer debriefing has taken place and that the researcher has taken a reflexive stance. However, it is most important that the authentic voices of the participants can be heard and that the findings present their life world or reality (as well as the voice of the researcher).

Findings and discussion

The findings must emerge directly from the data and their context. When researchers describe the findings after completion of the analysis, they link the description and themes they developed with the quotes of participants which demonstrate that the findings are grounded in the data. The discussion, which may or may not be integrated with the findings, engages actively with the literature connected to the findings.

The checklist

Many checklists have been written in the past about the evaluation of qualitative research. The following was developed for judging narrative inquiry. The structured approach to evaluation is not the only way to critically assess this type of research, but at least it gives some guidelines to do so. We have developed a list by which narrative research might be evaluated. Students or novice researchers might ask these questions of their own research. The evaluation list shares some of its features with the appraisal of all qualitative research.

Questions for evaluating a narrative study

The research question or problem
- Is the narrative approach suitable for this type of question or problem?
- Is the topic relevant and appropriate?
- Does the research focus on experience, thoughts and feelings of participants (rather than on the framework of the researcher)?
- Does it demand description or interpretation of subjective meanings of participants?

Research methodology and design
- How does it fit into the research philosophy or paradigm appropriate for narrative research?

- Are there good reasons for using narrative inquiry rather than other approaches?
- Does the researcher use the appropriate language for narrative research?
- Do the data have primacy (is the study inductive)?
- Is there a rationale for the strategies adopted?

The context
- Is there an appropriate description of the context of the research?
- Is the role of the researcher as 'research tool' clearly explained?

Ethical considerations
- Does the researcher explain general ethical issues as well as considering special features in the ethics of narrative research?
- Does the researcher describe ethical problems encountered and their solutions?
- Is there a statement about the need for ongoing consent?
- How are the data retrieved and kept?
- Has the researcher taken the appropriate steps for ethics committee approval?

Use of literature
- Does the initial review point to a gap in knowledge?
- Is the literature used in a non-directive way in the beginning?
- Does the researcher have an ongoing dialogue with the literature when discussing the findings?

Sampling
- Are the specifics of sampling in narrative inquiry explained?
- Does the researcher describe the type of sample as well as its limitations and inclusion and exclusion criteria?
- How did the researcher gain access to the participants?

Data collection and analysis
- Are the strategies for collecting and analysing data in place?
- Do the initial questions to the participant give guidance rather than direction?
- Is there minimal interference from the researcher throughout the storytelling?
- Are the participants in control of their stories?
- Is the analysis described in detail and with examples?

Validity or its alternatives
- Has the researcher explained trustworthiness (or validity) in a narrative study and how it differs from validity in quantitative research?

- Do the researchers describe how it has been achieved in their own study (through an audit trail, etc.)?

Findings and discussion
- Are the findings presented in accordance with the narrative approach?
- Does the researcher give excerpts from the words of the participants (quotes) to illustrate major points emerging in the findings?
- Is the discussion interwoven with the relevant literature which confirms or challenges the findings of the researcher?

The location and expertise of the researcher
- Have the researchers disclosed their own stance and location?
- Are they reflexive?
- Do they demonstrate familiarity with the narrative process?

Implications for nursing
- Are the implications for nursing apparent?
- Does this research contribute to practice?

Practical issues are not always considered by researchers as they are seen as trivial. The final narrative and report of the researchers, however, depends to some extent on how they have managed practicalities and solved problems in this arena. We shall now turn to the specific skills required to facilitate narrative interviews.

The skills of the narrative researcher

The skills of the narrative researcher include, but are not exclusively:

- Thinking narratively
- Reflexivity
- Self-awareness
- Developing empathy
- Permeability
- Move between reflection and action
- Continuity
- Communication
- Interaction
- Situatedness
- Connection
- Negotiation

Developing an empathic stance as researcher

Basic empathy enables the researcher to relate to the participant more completely, viewing the person as a whole rather than as an object. This more complete way of relating to the participant can be referred to as the I–Thou position (Buber, 1958). The incomplete experience of the self and other is known as the I–It attitude. As Briant and Freshwater (1998: 208) comment: 'The I–It attitude is one in which the other person is never viewed as a whole being. It can never be the basis for a holistic relationship.' The I–It position is one that has been found to exist widely within nursing. Menzies-Lyth (1970), in her research into social systems, found that nurses view patients as objects as a way of coping with the intense anxiety that such intimate relationships give rise to. The I–Thou approach to a relationship is based on equality, with one individual in their totality relating to the other in their totality. Given the social systems within which nurses have traditionally worked, an institutionalised I–It mode of operating is not surprising, but it does mean that nurse researchers have to think carefully about how they structure the research relationship, especially when conducting narrative inquiry. Although nurses generally possess the skills to create a therapeutic alliance, not all of them have translated this into the research encounter. Much of what takes places within narrative inquiry can be related to the person centred approach to nursing and caring.

Person centred relationships

Usually referred to as Rogerian counselling after its founder Carl Rogers, the person centred approach sits very much in the humanistic tradition. Rogers, influential as both a psychologist and a counsellor, became convinced during his career that human beings are essentially positive, forward looking and realistic by nature, which he referred to as the actualising tendency. Rogers believed this was the motivating force driving all human beings to achieve wholeness. When viewed from a humanistic perspective, nursing as a discipline can be seen as the ability to struggle with another through 'peak experiences related to health and suffering in which the participants in the nursing situation are and become in accordance with their human potential' (Paterson and Zderad, 1976: 7). Parse, a well known nursing theorist, captures this concept of 'potential' in her theory of health as human becoming (Parse, 1998), stating that the goal of the nurse living out the theory of human becoming is 'true presence in bearing witness and being with others in their changing health patterns' (Parse, 2001: 231).

Kleiman (2001: 167), an advocate of the humanistic approach to nursing, sees it as a call from humanity to maintain the humanness of the healthcare system, which she argues has become 'increasingly sophisticated in technology, increasingly concerned with cost containment, and increasingly less aware of and concerned with the patient as a human being'. We discussed the concept of managed care and the rise in technological nursing in an earlier chapter, but it is worth reminding the reader of the disillusionment of many nurses and healthcare professionals with the increasing dehumanisation of care. Similarly, nurse researchers have become dispirited by the objectification of the researcher–participant relationship. To truly realise patient centred care and participant centred research requires a commitment towards relationships that embraces the core conditions outlined by Carl Rogers (1961). It also means embracing the significant shift that we discussed in Chapter 3, from the medical model of cure to one of caring for the personhood of the client.

Creating the core conditions

Empathy

Empathy is a term that is employed variously in counselling, psychotherapy and nursing and across the helping professions. It is used to describe a particular characteristic that helpers should possess in relation to their clients. Here we are relating it to the skills of the narrative researcher, who will need to create a safe and enabling relationship to maximise both the potential of the data collection and the therapeutic potential of the storytelling for the participant. In broad terms empathy is a state of being between two people, where one is entering the world of the other while maintaining an awareness of his or her own world. It is the ability to see the world from the point of view of another individual, through their frame of reference, which in turn describes the ability of the helper to enter into the true feelings of the other person. It is not an attempt to be that person, rather to enter an imaginative state 'as if' one were that person, and try to envisage how it might feel to be them. It is the 'as if' quality that makes empathy different from sympathy. Sympathy, whilst concerned with feelings of pity, compassion and tenderness for the other person, involves collusion, whereas empathy requires much more effort, concentration and discipline.

Empathy is expressed or communicated through a number of key skills, including active listening to both the words and the feelings that are being conveyed by the participant. The reflecting back of the emotional content of the message from the storytellers in their own words enables them to feel that their message has been heard and understood. Basic empathy is associated with the beginnings of a helping relationship and the building of trust. Given the transient nature of research relationships, it is likely that the majority of encounters will be short lived, permitting usually a once-only interaction with the participant. However, relatively deep relationships are formed swiftly, where empathic responses are an important feature.

Genuineness and congruence

Basic empathy is dependent upon the researcher's warmth, genuineness and congruence. Sometimes referred to as genuineness, authenticity or transparency, congruence relates to the ability of the researcher to be a real person, that is to say that the researcher is not wedded to the idea of being the expert and does not assume a superior position in relation to the participant. This is often difficult to achieve within the context of nursing, not least because patients place nurses in the position of expert, expecting them to know more than they do.

There are also issues related to the power dynamics inherent within the nurse–patient/researcher–participant relationship.

Unconditional positive regard

Unconditional positive regard, sometimes referred to as acceptance, involves taking a non-judgemental stance towards the participants, accepting them and their story for who and what they are. Rogers (1991) was of the opinion that all individuals have a right to be accepted for who they are and that this sort of prizing of the person is necessary for them to feel safe. The key to achieving unconditional positive regard in any relationship is linked to the ability of the researcher/practitioner to differentiate between the person's behaviour and the person themselves. Thus within the person centred approach:

> 'the client's behaviour may be viewed as something quite separate from or even alien to him, since behaviour is, in any case, contingent upon the current circumstances or difficulties which the person is experiencing' (Hough, 1994: 34).

Nurses work with a diverse range of people from a wide range of social backgrounds, with differing beliefs and value systems around health. Many patients have risky health behaviours despite having information about the negative and potentially damaging aspects of their actions. Nurse researchers can sometimes hear difficult and challenging stories about individuals' behaviours and attitudes, which can make it hard for the researcher to remain engaged. Of course, it is possible that the researchers' and the participants' beliefs and values conflict altogether. In such complex situations working with a non-judgemental approach can prove problematic.

Creating an atmosphere of safety through the use of the core conditions is a fundamental aspect of the research relationship, enabling the expression of thoughts and feelings. Listening with a non-judgemental manner will encourage the participant to expand their awareness of themselves and their own personal narratives as well as ensuring the depth and richness of data collected. Although we are focusing on the participant as patient, the skills that we advocate are transferable across all research situations in narrative inquiry.

Establishing a rapport in the initial stages of the research relationship requires the skills of active listening, attention and attunement, genuine responses and empathy. Communication is what links us with other people and helps us to stay connected to society as a whole. There are many forms of communication; not all of them are speech related, indeed there are a range of non-verbal communication skills which can be used effectively to send and receive messages without the use of language. Where language is used, it can serve to make people feel either included or excluded and as such it is crucial that the narrative researcher is mindful of and reflects upon the language used by all parties involved.

Accurate listening

It is suggested that there are three phases to listening: receiving and understanding; communication of that understanding; and awareness in the other person that they have been heard and understood. MacLeod Clark et al. (1992) further describe the levels of listening as listening for facts, for feelings and for intentions. In *Swift to Hear*, Jacobs (2000) provides guidelines for listening which are useful in raising awareness of what *not* to do when attempting to establish a bond with participants. Freshwater (2003) notes that the skills of active and accurate listening include:

- Reflecting meaning
- Reflecting feeling
- Silence
- Questioning
- Paraphrasing
- Summarising
- Ability to listen to oneself

Using these skills enables the patient to hear their thoughts and feelings aloud in the context of storytelling. Listening, however, is not just about hearing the words of the speaker; it is also about observing the use of body language, both the participant's and one's own. Appropriate use of eye contact, for example, can be used to communicate that the researcher is willing to engage. Voice tone, pace and pitch can also do much to change the atmosphere of a situation. Researchers can indicate with their body language that they are attending, by nodding, by facing the narrator, by leaning forward and by using an open body posture. Distractions to active accurate listening can be both internal (within the researcher) and external (the setting, noises, other pressing priorities).

Reflecting meaning

Reflecting back what a person has said is widely used in all types of communication, letting the narrator know that the listener has understood the key message. This can take the form of a question, or of selective 'echoing', and can be used to highlight crucial words or points. For example, a participant being interviewed about discharge planning following surgery might say 'I really wasn't sure if I was ready to go home when the nurse came to help me pack my things. In fact, I really felt unprepared.' The researcher might respond by simply saying 'You didn't feel prepared to go home?' in the form of a question, encouraging the narrator to be more explicit: 'Yes, actually I only found out two hours beforehand and I didn't think I would be going home for another two days . . .'. Selective echoing encourages the participants to expand upon their earlier statement.

Reflecting feeling

The aim of reflecting feelings is to focus attention on the feeling aspect of a narrative rather than on the content alone, since it can help to raise awareness of vague unexpressed feelings that are not easily acknowledged, but are important in the context of the narrative. Reflecting back feelings can sometimes elicit cathartic expressions of strong emotions, particularly in situations where distress has been contained for some time. Indeed, the skill of simple reflection has the potential to be a powerful facilitative intervention; even though the participants might have powerful reactions, they might still experience a sense of relief at feeling the emotion and having it witnessed.

Listening to self

Burnard (1992: 000) writes of the importance of staying awake whilst listening! He goes on to say that 'it is vital that people *notice* their own feelings and thoughts, their own body position, posture, eye contact and so forth'. Staying awake in this way means being more observant and attuned both to the needs of others and to one's own needs. This developing sense of self-awareness may at first lead to the experience of self-consciousness. Learning new skills, or making previously taken for granted skills more conscious, invariably creates a degree of self-consciousness, causing some embarrassment and shyness (Freshwater, 2003). Self-consciousness gradually transforms into a continual process of noticing and examining aspects of the self with the purpose of deepening personal and interpersonal understanding.

Self-awareness has been widely written about in nursing and in research circles. It has gained huge momentum over recent years alongside increasing awareness of reflective practice and reflexivity in research. Self-awareness in research can help the researcher:

- To make decisions on the most appropriate responses
- To assess their personal abilities, limitations and training requirements
- To obtain feedback on personal performance during skilled action

The process of becoming self-aware is both an introspective one and one which requires feedback from other people. Narrative researchers can elicit feedback from a number of sources, from supervisors to peers and of course the storytellers themselves.

Silence

Silence, a rarity in human communication and, it seems, contemporary society, particularly within busy healthcare settings, is a skill that provides a different experience for the patient as participant. Silence can be a resting place for participants and researchers, a time when reflection can take place. But it is not easy to tolerate. Whilst silence may encourage the storyteller to talk, it might also incite the researcher to interject and fill the empty space. Freshwater (2003) categorises silences in the following way:

- Passive
- Active
- Creative
- Destructive

Positive silences, characterised by intimacy and harmony, feel comfortable and they encourage all parties to become more aware of their inner worlds and of each other. In this sense the silence is active *and* creative. Negative silences are less comfortable and are associated with a tension that suggests animosity or hostility. If the researcher is unsure how to progress in the silence, a simple 'What's happening?' or 'What are you feeling at this moment?' offers the participant the opportunity to say as much or as little about the silence as they feel able to. Freshwater and Robertson (2002) provide an example of the complexity of silence as narrated by a therapist:

'There is often silence between us and it has different nuances depending on what is happening or not happening in the relationship. There are warm silences when the empathic resonance is strong. Sometimes these feel like a warm bath, cleansing and relaxing, it holds and radiates a soft heat. We feel close and intimate. She is able to say very difficult things in the confidence of being received. The heat is probably provided by Eros but he is not charging things up, just allowing his presence to warm us.

Other times the silences are cool. They stretch the distance between us and I have to make a great effort to reach across with my words which often seem to languish by the way and never reach their destination. This coolness is not the same as a frozen or icy state in which fear and hate predominate. It is more to do with the absence of emotion or need, a detachment that somehow insulates us from each other. I notice the coolness not so much from the expression of any particular verbal or non-verbal communication. It is more in the absence of a reciprocal affinity that we have built together. In this affinity we are attuned, without it there isn't any music for us to attune to. So it is not even a question of being out of tune. The coolness could be thought of as a detachment but even this is too concrete. It is an expression of what is missing.'

Open-ended prompts

Prompts can be used to encourage the participants to continue speaking and may include non-verbal encouragement such as nodding, or verbal prompts such as echoing the last word or phrase said. Other prompts include 'Yes', 'Go on', 'And then . . .'. Silence can also be used as a prompt, encouraging a train of thought without interruption.

Questioning

Questions are verbal communications which initiate particular responses and can be used in a variety of ways to open channels of communication. Questions can be *questioner centred, participant focused* and *group activity*. The first type are used mainly to meet the need of the questioner, and may be employed to obtain information, to focus attention, to arouse or spark off interest and curiosity and to initiate social interaction. Hence, the narrative researcher may begin the interview with a questioner centred question. However, the same question might also be participant focused, aiming to discover facts about the narrators and taking a genuine interest in them.

Questions, used with intention and deliberation, provide numerous opportunities to deepen and enhance the research relationship, prompting the participants to go further with their exploration. Questions can also have a catalytic potential, helping to draw out the reluctant or reticent participant in a facilitative manner. Nevertheless, they can also be overused and used in an interrogative manner, thereby creating a barrier.

Open questions

Open questions do not suggest or require a predetermined response, and permit the respondent the freedom to answer in a number of ways. They are particularly useful in narrative research for exploring personal information. Open questions usually begin with *how, when, where,* or *what* and are generally formulated in broad terms so as to initiate a flow of information. They can be advantageous in that very little prior knowledge is required to formulate the question and yet a great deal of unexpected data can be elicited.

Closed questions

Asking closed questions limits the type of response that can be made, usually eliciting a simple but less than informative 'Yes' or 'No' answer. More often than not closed questions are used to ascertain factual information, with the content and the response being dictated by the questioner (questioner centred). Further types of closed questions are the selective question, in which the answer to the question is restricted by providing the storyteller with a few alternatives, and the factual question. Factual closed questions are used frequently in nursing but are not particularly helpful in narrative research except where simple answers to factual questions are required.

Probing questions

This type of question encourages expansion on previously made points. Probing questions may help in clarifying a problem and in eliciting examples of specific issues: 'Can you give an example of what might trigger off the panic attacks?'

Affective questions

Affective questions ask the respondent to relate their feelings, referring to the subjective emotional state of the individual as opposed to the objective interpretation of facts.

Rhetorical questions

Rhetorical questions are not asked with the intention of receiving an answer: indeed at times the questioner may go on to provide the answer themselves, or use the question as a summary, before moving the storyteller on by asking a further question.

Reciprocity and dialogue

During narrative interviews a self-consciousness develops as the relationship tends towards the I–Thou encounter. Both researcher and participant become subjects of discovery as opposed to objects of examination [for a more in-depth analysis of the I–It, I–Thou modes of relating see Martin Buber (1958)]. The deepening connection with the researcher enables the narrator to experiment with the expression of feelings and to explore needs and to begin to develop a sense of him- or herself as a separate person. Such self-awareness can often bring the sense of 'thinking about thinking' to the research situation, or thinking narratively.

Both Barton (2004) and Lindsay and Smith (2003) write about 'thinking narratively'. One could question whether one has to have a specific type of thinking to be a narrative researcher, for surely we are all narrators of our lives and storytellers? Perhaps we need to become more aware of those skills and then use them intentionally and with purpose. Thinking narratively means moving between the present and the past, working with memories across time and space in a circular rather than linear pattern. Clandinin and Connelly (2000) suggest that narrative is three-dimensional and not something that happens alone. Narrative happens in an interactive space, one in which co-construction of identities takes place and where individuals meet.

According to Buber (1958: 25): 'all real living is meeting'. The currency of this meeting is dialogue. Dialogue is not just about verbal and non-verbal interaction, but much more, as the physicist and cosmologist David Bohm (1990) notes in his work on wholeness and dialogue. These are not unfamiliar concepts to nursing; a person's experience of herself or himself in this world is through psychological and physiological awareness, contained within a reflexive dialogue with both the self and the outside world. Cole (2001: 11) argues that:

> The presence of dialogue offers the *possibility* of balance, a state of equilibrium, a stress-less state. But the nature of the dialogue determines whether there is actually a balance, a state without stress, or whether a lack of balance indicates a state of stress.

The significant part of this statement in the current context is 'the nature of the dialogue'. If the nature of the dialogue is empathic, then this is confirming and grounding for both the narrator and the researcher.

Summary

We have discussed the practical aspects of narrative inquiry such as tape recording and transcription and the ways in which researchers can evaluate their own and others' work. However, there are some issues that are even more important. As we have reiterated throughout this book, narrative research is about relationships, with both clients and colleagues; as such, narrative researchers need to develop self-awareness and interpersonal and emotional skills to cope with the sometimes difficult nature of the work. Such skills can be developed within the context of reflective practice, research supervision, and other dialogical forums.

Creating and maintaining a climate within which the skills of empathic dialogue can be used effectively is an essential part of the narrative process. Both directive and non-directive skills may be appropriate to use within the narrative encounter. However, the emphasis of a non-directive approach is on the person and their natural capacity to come to terms with and solve their own problems through telling their story.

References

Abma T.A. (1999) Powerful stories: the role of stories in sustaining and transforming professional practice with a mental hospital. In: Josselson R. & Lieblich A. (Eds) *Interpreting Experience: The Narrative Study of Lives*, pp. 169–196. Thousand Oaks, Sage.

Albarran J.W. & Scholes J. (2005) How to get published: seven easy steps. *Nursing in Critical Care* **10** (2), 72–77.

Altheide D.L. & Johnson J.M. (1994) Criteria for assessing interpretive validity in qualitative research. In: Denzin N.K. & Lincoln Y.S. (Eds) *Handbook of Qualitative Research*, pp. 465–499. Thousand Oaks, Sage.

Alvermann D.E. (2000) Narrative approaches. *Reading Online* **4** (5). http://www.readingonline.org/articles/art_index.asp?HREF=/articles/handbook/alvermann/index.hmtl

Anderson J.M. (1991) Reflexivity in fieldwork: toward a feminist epistemology. *Image: Journal of Nursing Scholarship* **23** (2), 115–118.

Androutsopoulou A. (2001) Fiction as an aid to therapy: a narrative and family rationale for practice. *Journal of Family Therapy* **23**, 278–295.

Aranda S. & Street A. (2000) From individual to group: use of narratives in a participatory research process. *Journal of Advanced Nursing* **33** (6), 791–797.

Archakis A. & Tzanne A. (2005) Narrative positioning and the construction of situated identities. *Narrative Inquiry* **15** (2), 267–291.

Atkinson P.A. (1997) Narrative turn or blind alley? *Qualitative Health Research* **7** (3), 325–344.

Atkinson P. & Silverman D. (1997) Kundera's immortality: the interview society and the invention of the self. *Qualitative Inquiry* **3** (3), 304–325.

Atkinson P., Coffey A. & Delamont S. (2003) *Key Themes in Qualitative Research: Continuities and Change*. Walnut Creek, Altamira Press.

Bakhtin M.M. (1981) *The Dialogic Imagination*. Austin, University of Texas Press.

Baldwin C. (2004) Narrative analysis and contested allegations of Munchausen syndrome by proxy. In: Hurwitz B., Greenhalgh T. & Skultans V. (Eds) *Narrative Research in Health and Illness*. Oxford, Blackwell Publishing, BMJ Books.

Barbour R.S. (2003) The newfound credibility of qualitative research? Tales of technical essentialism and co-option. *Qualitative Health Research* **13** (7), 1019–1027.

Barthes R. (1982) *Introduction to the Structural Analysis of Narratives. A Barthes Reader*. New York, Hill and Wang.

Bartol G. (1989) Creative literature: an aid to nursing practice. *Nursing and Health Care* **10** (8), 453–457.

Barton S.S. (2004) Narrative inquiry: locating aboriginal epistemology in a relational methodology. *Journal of Advanced Nursing* **45** (5), 519–526.

Becker B. (2001) Challenging 'ordinary' pain: narratives of older people who live with pain. In: Kenyon G., Clark P. & deVries B. (Eds) *Narrative Gerontology: Theory, Research and Practice*, pp. 91–112. Springer, New York.

Begley A. (1996) Literature and poetry: pleasure and practice. *International Journal of Nursing Practice* **2**, 182–188.

Benner P. (1984) *From Novice to Expert.* Menlo Park, Addison Wesley.

Bircumshaw D. (1990) The utilization of research findings in clinical nursing practice. *Journal of Advanced Nursing* **15**, 1272–1280.

Bird P. (1994) The poetry of nursing. *Clinical Nurse Specialist* **8** (6), 293–295.

Bishop V. & Freshwater D. (2003) Conducting research in a clinical environment: research methods, questions and support. In: Freshwater D. & Bishop V. (Eds) *Nursing Research in Context.* Basingstoke, Palgrave Macmillan.

Blackmore S. (2001) State of the art: consciousness. *The Psychologist* **14** (10), 522–525.

Blumenreich M. (2004) Avoiding the pitfalls of 'conventional' narrative research: Using post-structural theory to guide the creation of narratives of children with HIV. *Qualitative Research* **4** (1), 77–90.

Bohm D. (1990) *On Dialogue.* London, Routledge.

Bonnell C. (1999) Evidence based nursing: a stereotyped view of quantitative and experimental research could work against professional autonomy and authority. *Journal of Advanced Nursing* **30** (1), 18–23.

Borland K. (1991) 'That's not what I said': interpretive conflict in oral narrative research. In: Gluck S.B. & Patai D. (Eds) *Women's Words.* London, Routledge.

Boykin A. & Schoenhofer S. (1990) Caring in nursing: analysis of extant theory. *Nursing Science Quarterly* **3**, 149–155.

Braud W.G. (1994) Honouring our natural experiences. *Journal of the American Society for Psychical Research* **88** (3), 293–308.

Braud W. & Anderson R. (1998) *Transpersonal Research Methods for the Social Sciences.* London, Sage.

Briant S. & Freshwater D. (1998) Exploring mutuality within the nurse–patient relationship. *British Journal of Nursing* **7** (4), 204–211.

Brody H. (2003) *Stories of Sickness*, 2nd edn. New York, Oxford University Press.

Bruner J. (1986) *Actual Minds, Possible Words.* Cambridge, Harvard University Press.

Bruner J. (1991) The narrative construction of reality. *Critical Inquiry* **18**, 1–21.

Bruner J. (2002) *Making Stories: Law, Literature, Life.* New York, Farrar, Strauss and Giroux.

Brykczynska G. (1997) Art and literature: nursing's distant mirror? In: Brykczynska G. (Ed.) *Caring: The Compassion and Wisdom of Nursing.* London, Arnold.

Bryman A. (2001) *Social Research Methods.* Oxford, Oxford University Press.

Bryman A. (2006) Editorial. *Qualitative Research* **6** (1), 5–7.

Buber M. (1970) *I and Thou*, 2nd edn. Edinburgh, T. & T. Clark.

Burnard P. (1992) Learning from experience: the nurse tutors' and student nurses' perceptions of experiential learning in nurse education: some initial findings. *International Journal of Nursing Studies* **29** (2), 151–161.

Bury M. (2001) Illness narratives: fact or fiction? *Sociology of Health and Illness* **23** (3), 263–285.

Butler J. (1993) *Bodies that Matter: On the Discursive Limits of Sex.* London, Routledge.

Canadian Task Force on the Periodic Health Examination (1979) The Periodic Health Examination. *Canadian Medical Health Association Journal* **121**, 1139–1254.

Capasso V. (1998) The theory is in the practice: an exemplar. *Clinical Nurse Specialist* **12** (6), 226–229.

Carper B. (1978) Fundamental patterns of knowing. *Advances in Nursing Science* **1**, 13–24.

Casement P. (1985) *On Learning from the Patient*. London, Tavistock.

Chamberlayne P., Bornat J. & Wengraf T. (2000) *The Turn to Biographical Methods in Social Science*. London, Routledge.

Charmaz K. (1999) Stories of suffering: subjective tales and research narratives. *Qualitative Health Research* **9** (3), 362–383.

Chatman S. (1978) *Story and Discourse: Narrative Structure in Fiction and Film*. London, Cornell University Press.

Chiarella M. (2000) Silence in court: the devaluation of the stories of nurses in the narratives of health law. *Nursing Inquiry* **7** (3), 191–199.

Chinn P.L. & Kramer M.K. (1995) *Theory and Nursing: A Systematic Approach*, 4th edition. St Louis, C.V. Mosby.

Chinn P.L. & Watson J. (1994) *Art and Aesthetics in Nursing*. New York, National League for Nursing Press.

Churchill S.D. (2000) 'Seeing through' self-deception in narrative reports: finding psychological truth in problematic data. *Journal of Phenomenological Psychology* **31** (1), 44–62.

Clandinin J.D. & Connelly M.F. (2000) *Narrative Inquiry: Experience and Story in Qualitative Research*. San Francisco, Jossey Bass.

Clarkson P. (1989) *Gestalt Counselling in Action*. London, Sage.

Closs J. & Cheater F.M. (1999) Evidence for nursing practice: a clarification of the issues. *Journal of Advanced Nursing* **30** (1), 10–17.

Cobley P. (2004) *Narrative*. London, Routledge.

Coffey A., Holbrook B. & Atkinson P. (1996) Qualitative data analysis: technologies and representations. *Sociological Research Online*. http://www.socreonline.org.uk/socreonline/1/1/4.html.

Cohan S. & Shires L.M. (1988) *Telling Stories: A Theoretical Analysis of Narrative Fiction*. London, Routledge.

Cole S. (2001) A place for person centred therapy. *Health Care Counselling and Psychotherapy Journal* **1** (1), 14–17.

Colyer H. & Kamath P. (1999) Evidence based practice. A philosophical and political analysis: some matters for consideration by professional practitioners. *Journal of Advanced Nursing* **29** (1), 188–193.

Connelly M. & Clandinin J. (1990) Stories of experience and narrative inquiry. *Educational Researcher* **19** (5), 2–14.

Cortazzi M. (1993) *Narrative Analysis*. London, Falmer Press.

Couser G.T. (1997) *Recovering Bodies: Illness, Disability and Life Writing*. Madison, University of Wisconsin Press.

Creswell J.W. (2003) *Research Design: Qualitative, Quantitative and Mixed Method Approaches*, 2nd edn. Thousand Oaks, Sage.

Czarniawska B. (2004) *Narratives in Social Research*. London, Sage.

Dahlberg K. (2006) The publication of qualitative research findings. *Qualitative Health Research* **16** (3), 444–446.

Dahlberg K., Drew N. & Nyström M. (2001) *Reflective Lifeworld Research*. Lund, SE, Studentlitteratur.

Darbyshire P. (1995) In defence of pedagogy: a critique of the notion of andragogy. *Nurse Education Today* **13**, 328–335.

Davies D. & Dodd J. (2002) Qualitative research and the question of rigor. *Qualitative Health Research* **12** (2), 279–289.

Davis R. & Shadle M. (2000) 'Building a mystery': alternative research writing and the academic act of seeking. *College Composition and Communication* **51** (3), 417–446.

Dawson G. (1994) *Soldier Heroes*. Routledge.

Daymon C. & Holloway I. (2002) *Qualitative Research for Public Relations and Marketing Communications*. London, Routledge.

Day-Sclater S. (1998) Creating the self: stories as transitional phenomena. *Autobiography* **VI**, 85–92.

Dean J.F. & Whyte W.E. (1958) How do you know if the informant is telling the truth? *Human Organization* **17**, 34–38.

Denzin N.K. (1989) *Interpretive Biography*. Beverly Hills, Sage.

Denzin N.K. (2001) The reflexive interview and a performative social science. *Qualitative Research* **1** (1), 23–46.

DH (Department of Health) (1998) *Modernising social services, promoting independence, improving protection, raising standards* (Cm 4169). London, The Stationery Office (TSO).

DH (2000) *The NHS Plan: a plan for investment, a plan for reform* (Cm 4818). London, TSO.

DHSS (1983) *Inquiry into NHS Management (The Griffiths Report)*. London, HMSO.

Donald A. (1998) The words we live in. In: Greenhalgh T. and Hurwitz B. (1998) *Narrative Based Medicine*. London, BMJ Books.

Elliott J. (2005) *Using Narrative in Social Research: Qualitative and Quantitative Approaches*. London, Sage.

Erlandson D.A., Harris E.L., Skipper B.L. & Allen S.D. (1993) *Doing Naturalistic Inquiry: A Guide to Methods*. Newbury Park, Sage.

Ewick P. & Silbey S.S. (1995) Subversive stories and hegemonic tales: toward a sociology of narrative. *Law and Society Review* **29** (2), 197–226.

Finch J. (1984) It's great to have someone to talk to: the ethics and politics of interviewing women. In: Bell C. & Roberts H. (Eds) *Social Researching*. London, Routledge and Kegan Paul.

Forster E.M. (1927) *Aspects of the Novel*. London, Penguin.

Fossey E., Harvey C., McDermott F. & Davidson L. (2002) Understanding and evaluating qualitative research. *Australian and New Zealand Journal of Psychiatry* **36**, 717–732.

Frank A.W. (1995) *The Wounded Storyteller: Body, Illness and Ethics*. Chicago, Chicago University Press.

Frank A.W. (2000) The standpoint of the storyteller. *Qualitative Health Research* **10** (3), 354–365.

Frank A.W. (2002) An overview of narrative analysis. Narrative Workshop 2. *Qualitative Research Conference*, Banff.

Freeman M. (2003) Identity and difference in narrative inquiry: a commentary on the articles by Erica Burman, Michelle Crossley, Ian Parker and Shelley Slater. *Narrative Inquiry* **13** (2), 331–346.

French P. (1999) The development of evidence based nursing. *Journal of Advanced Nursing* **29** (1), 72–78.

Freshwater D. (1998) Transformatory Learning in Nurse Education. Unpublished PhD Thesis, University of Nottingham.

Freshwater D. (2000) *Transformational Learning through Reflective Practice*. Portsmouth, Nursing Praxis International.

Freshwater D. (Ed.) (2002) *Therapeutic Nursing: Improving Patient Care through Self-awareness and Reflection*. London, Sage.

Freshwater D. (2003) Pathology in a post modern society. *NTResearch* **8** (3), 161–172.

Freshwater D. (2004) Emotional intelligence: developing emotionally literate training in mental health. *Mental Health Practice* **8** (4), 12–15.

Freshwater D. (2006) Reflective practice and clinical supervision: two sides of the same coin. In: Bishop V. (Ed.) *Clinical Supervision*. Basingstoke, Palgrave.

Freshwater D. & Avis M. (2004) Analysing interpretation and reinterpreting analysis. *Nursing Philosophy* **5**, 4–11.

Freshwater D. & Robertson C. (2002) *Emotions and Needs*. Buckingham, Open University Press.

Freshwater D. & Rolfe G. (2004) *Deconstructing Evidence Based Practice*. London, Routledge.

Freshwater D. & Stickley T. (2003) The heart of the art: emotional intelligence in nurse education. *Nursing Inquiry* **11** (2), 91–98.

Freud S. (1915) *The Unconscious*, standard edn, Vol. 12. London, Hogarth Press.

Frey B.S. (2003) Publishing as prostitution? – choosing between one's own ideas and academic success. *Public Choice* **116**, 205–223.

Frid I., Öhlsen J. & Bergbom I. (2000) On the use of narratives in nursing research. *Journal of Advanced Nursing* **32** (3), 695–703.

Gallagher S. & Shear J. (Ed.) (1999) *Models of the Self*. Exeter, Imprint Academic.

Galvin K., Todres L. & Richardson M. (2005) The intimate mediator: a carer's experience of Alzheimer's. *Scandinavian Journal of Caring Science* **19**, 2–11.

Garro L.C. (1994) Narrative representations of chronic illness experience: cultural models of illness, mind and body in stories concerning the temporomandibular joint (TMJ). *Social Science and Medicine* **38** (6), 775–788.

Garro L.C. (2000) Cultural knowledge as resource in illness narratives: remembering through accounts of illness. In: Mattingly C. & Garro L.C. (Eds) *Narrative and the Cultural Construction of Illness and Healing*, pp. 70–87. Berkeley, University of California Press.

Geertz C. (1973) *The Interpretation of Cultures*. New York, Basic Books.

Geertz C. (1994) Thick description: toward an interpretive theory of culture. In: McIntyre M. (Ed.) *Readings in the Philosophy of Social Science*, pp. 213–231. Cambridge, Cambridge University Press.

Gergen K.J. & Gergen M.M. (1987) Narratives of the self. In: Hinchman L.P. and Hinchman S.K. (Eds) *Memory, Identity and Community: The Idea of Narrative in the Human Sciences*. New York, State University of New York.

Gergen K.J. & Gergen M. (1988) Narrative and the self as relationship. In: Berkowitz L. (Ed.) *Advances in Social Psychology*, Vol. 21, pp. 17–56. San Diego, Academic Press.

Gergen M.M. & Gergen K.J. (2003) Qualitative inquiry: tensions and transformations. In: Denzin N.K. & Lincoln Y.S. (Eds) *The Landscape of Qualitative Research: Theories and Issues*, 2nd edn. London, Sage.

Gilgun J.F. (2005) 'Grab' and good science: writing up the results of qualitative research. *Qualitative Health Research* **15** (2), 256–262.

Glaser B.G. (1978) *Theoretical Sensitivity.* Mill Valley, Sociology Press.

Glaser B.G. (1999) The future of grounded theory. Keynote address from the Fourth Annual Qualitative Health Research Conference. *Qualitative Health Research* **9** (6), 836–845.

Goncalves O.F., Henriques M.R. & Machado P.P.P. (2004) Nurturing narrative. In: Angus L.E. and McLeod J. (Eds) *The Handbook of Narrative and Psychotherapy: Practice, Theory and Research.* London, Sage.

Graham H. (1984) Surveying through stories. In: C. Bell and H. Roberts (Ed.) *Social Researching: Politics, Problems, Practice.* London, Routledge and Kegan Paul.

Greenhalgh T. & Hurwitz B. (1998) Why study narrative? In: Greenhalgh T. & Hurwitz B. (Eds) *Narrative Based Medicine: Dialogue and Discourse in Clinical Practice,* pp. 3–16. London, BMJ Books.

Greenhalgh T., Russell J. & Swinglehurst D. (2005) Narrative methods in quality improvement research. *Quality and Safety in Health Care* **14** (6), 443–449.

Greenwood J. (1984) Nursing research: a position paper. *Journal of Advanced Nursing* **9**, 77–82.

Guba E.G. & Lincoln Y.S. (1989) *Fourth Generation Evaluation.* Newbury Park, Sage.

Gudmundsdottir S. (1998) How to turn interpretative research into a narrative. Research Seminar Narrative – biographical methods in research on teachers and teaching. Oulu, Finland.

Häninnen V. (2004) A model of narrative circulation. *Narrative Inquiry* **14** (1), 69–85.

Haraway D. (1988) Situated knowledge. *Feminist Studies* **14**, 575–599.

Harding S. (1992) *Whose Science? Whose Knowledge?* Milton Keynes, Open University Press.

Harré R. (2004) Staking our claim for qualitative psychology as science. *Research in Psychology* **1** (1), 3–14.

Hart C. (1998) *Doing a Literature Review.* London, Sage.

Hartsock N.C.M. (1997) *The Feminist Standpoint Revisited.* New York, Basic Books.

Harvey G., Kitson A.L. & McCormack B. (1997) Approaches to implementing research in practice. *Second European Forum on Quality in Health Care*, Palais de Congres, Paris, 24–26 April.

Holloway I. (1997) *Basic Concepts for Qualitative Research.* Oxford, Blackwell Science.

Holloway I. (2005) Qualitative writing. In: Holloway I. (Ed.) *Qualitative Research in Health Care,* pp. 288–304. Maidenhead, Open University Press.

Holloway I. & Walker J. (2000) *Getting a PhD in Health and Social Care.* Oxford, Blackwell Science.

Holloway I. & Wheeler S. (2002) *Qualitative Research in Nursing.* Oxford, Blackwell.

Holloway I., Sofaer B. & Walker J. (2000) The transition from well person to 'pain afflicted' patient: the career of people with chronic back pain. *Illness, Crisis and Loss* **8** (4), 373–387.

Hollway W. & Jefferson T. (2000) *Doing Qualitative Research Differently.* London, Sage.

Holstein J. & Gubrium J. (1995) *The Active Interview.* Thousand Oaks, Sage.

Hopkins A. (1992) *Measures of the Quality of Life and the Uses to which Such Measures May be Put.* London, Royal College of Physicians.

Hough M. (1994) *A Practical Approach to Counselling*. London, Pitman.

Howarth A. (2006) The experience of aromatherapy massage for patients diagnosed with multiple sclerosis and chronic pain. Unpublished PhD Thesis, Bournemouth University.

Hughson E.A. & Brown R.I. (1988) The evaluation of rehabilitation programmes. *Irish Journal of Psychology* **9** (2), 249–263.

Hunter K.M. (1991) *Doctors' Stories: The Narrative Structure of Medical Knowledge*. Princeton, Princeton University Press.

Hunter K.M. (1996) Narrative, literature and the clinical exercise of practical reason. *Journal of Medical Philosophy* **21**, 303–320.

Hurwitz B., Greenhalgh T. & Skultans V. (Eds) (2004) *Narrative Research in Health and Illness*. Oxford, BMJ Books/Blackwell Publishing.

Hyvärinen M. (2004) The conceptual history of narrative: an outline. Conference in Helsinki, 3–4 December.

Jacobs M. (2000) *Swift to Hear: Facilitating Skills in Listening and Responding*. London, New Library of Pastoral Care, SPCK Publishing.

Järvinen M. (2004) Life history and the perspective of the present. *Narrative Inquiry* **14** (1), 45–68.

Johnson J. (1994) A dialectical examination of nursing art. *Advances in Nursing Science* **17**, 1–14.

Johnson L.J. (1996) Nursing art and prescriptive truths. In: Kikuchi J.F., Simmons H. & Romyn D. (Eds) *Truth in Nursing Inquiry*, pp. 36–50. Thousand Oaks, Sage.

Jonas C.M. (1994) True presence through music. *Nursing Science Quarterly* **103** (3), 112–114.

Jones A.H. (1990) Literature and medicine: traditions and innovations. In: Clarke B. & Aycock W. (Eds) *The Body and the Text: Comparative Essays in Literature and Medicine*. Lubbock, Texas Technical University Press.

Jones K. (2005a) The art of collaborative storytelling: arts-based representations of narrative contexts. Draft for: International Sociological Research Committee on Biography and Society. RC38 Newsletter.

Jones K. (2005b) Developing a performative social science for qualitative researchers. Master Class, Bournemouth University, October.

Jones R.A. (2005) Identity commitments in personal stories of mental illness on the internet. *Narrative Inquiry* **15** (2), 293–322.

Josselson R. & Lieblich A. (Eds) (1993) *The Narrative Study of Lives*, Vol. 1. Newbury Park, Sage.

Josselson R. & Lieblich A. (Eds) (1995) *Interpreting Experience: The Narrative Study of Lives*. Thousand Oaks, Sage.

Josselson R. & Lieblich A. (2001) Narrative research and humanism. In: Schneider K.J., Bugental F.T. & Pierson J.F. *The Handbook of Humanistic Psychology: Leading Edges in Theory, Research, and Practice*, pp. 275–288. Thousand Oaks, Sage.

Jovchelovitch S. & Bauer M.W. (2000) Narrative interviewing. In: M.W. Bauer & G. Gaskell (Eds) *Qualitative Interviewing with Text, Image and Sound*. London, Sage.

Katims I. (1993) Nursing as aesthetic experience and the notion of practice. *Scholarly Inquiry for Nursing Practice: An International Journal* **7** (4), 269–278.

Keen S. & Todres L. (2006) Communicating qualitative research findings: an annotated bibliographic review of non-traditional dissemination strategies. Report, Bournemouth University.

Kellas J.K. & Manusov V. (2003) What's in a story? The relationship between narrative completeness and adjustment to relationship dissolution. *Journal of Social and Personal Relationships* **20** (3), 285–307.

Kikuchi J.F. & Simmons H. (1996) The whole truth and progress in nursing development. In: Kikuchi J.F., Simmons H. & Romyn D. (Eds) *Truth in Nursing Inquiry*, pp. 5–18. Thousand Oaks, Sage.

Kitson A. (1997) Using evidence to demonstrate the value of nursing. *Nursing Standard* **11** (28), 34–39.

Kleiman S. (2001) Josephine Paterson and Loretta Zderad. Humanistic nursing theory with clinical applications. In: Parker M. (Ed.) *Nursing Theories and Nursing Practice*. Philadelphia, F. A. Davis.

Klein J. (1987) *Our Need for Others and Its Roots in Infancy*. Tavistock, London.

Kleinman A. (1988) *The Illness Narratives: Suffering, Healing and the Human Condition*. New York, Basic Books.

Kleinman A. (1996) *Writing at the Margin: Discourse between Anthropology and Medicine*. Berkeley, University of California Press.

Kreiswirth R. (2000) Merely telling stories: narrative knowing and the human sciences. *Poetics Today* **21** (2), 291–318.

Kvale S. (1996) *InterViews: An Introduction to Qualitative Research Interviewing*. Thousand Oaks, Sage.

Labkowicz N. (1967) *Theory and Practice*. Lanham, University Press of America.

Labov W. & Waletzky J. (1967) Narrative analysis: oral versions of personal experience. In: Helm J. (Ed.) *Essays on the Verbal and Visual Arts*, pp. 12–44. Seattle, University of Washington Press.

Labov W. & Waletzky J. (1997) Oral versions of personal experience: three decades of narrative analysis. *Journal of Narrative and Life History* **7**, 3–38.

Le May A., Mulhall A. & Alexander C. (1998) Bridging the research–practice gap: exploring the research cultures of practitioners and managers. *Journal of Advanced Nursing* **28** (2), 428–437.

Lieblich A. (1996) Some unforeseen outcomes of conducting narrative research with people of one's own culture. In Josselson R. (Ed.) *Ethics and Process in the Narrative Study of Lives*. Thousand Oaks, Sage.

Lieblich A., Tuval-Mashiach R. & Zilber T. (1998) *Narrative Research: Reading, Analysis and Interpretation*. Thousand Oaks, Sage.

Lincoln Y. & Guba E. (1985) *Naturalistic Inquiry*. Thousand Oaks, Sage.

Lindsay G.M. & Smith F. (2003) Narrative inquiry in a nursing practicum. *Nursing Inquiry* **10** (2), 121–129.

Locke L.F., Spirduso W.W. & Silverman S.J. (2000) *Proposals that Work*, 4th edition. Thousand Oaks, Sage.

Long A.F. (1998) Health services research – a radical approach to cross the research and development divide. In: Baker M. & Kirk S. (Eds) *Research and Development for the NHS*. Oxford, Radcliffe Medical Press.

Lucas J. (1997) Making sense of interviews: the narrative dimension. *Social Sciences in Health* **3** (2), 113–126.

Lupton D. (1994) *Medicine as Culture: Illness, Disease and the Body in Western Societies*. London, Sage.

MacLeod Clark J., Kendall S. & Haverty S. (1992) Effective use of health education skills. In: Horne E. & Cowan T. (Eds) *Effective Communication: Nursing Perspectives*. London, Wolfe.

Maeve M.K. (1994) The carrier bag theory of nursing practice. *Advances in Nursing Science* **4** (9), 9–22.

Marks-Maran D. (1999) Reconstructing nursing: evidence, artistry and the curriculum. *Nurse Education Today* **19**, 3–11.

Mason J. (2002) *Qualitative Researching*, 2nd edn. London, Sage.

Maxwell J.A. (2004, March). Causal explanation, qualitative research, and scientific inquiry in education. *Educational Researcher*, **33** (2), 3–11.

McClarey M. & Duff L. (1997) Clinical effectiveness and evidence based practice. *Nursing Standard* **11** (52), 33–37.

McKenzie R. (2002) The importance of philosophical congruence for therapeutic use of self in practice. In: Freshwater D. (Ed.) *Therapeutic Nursing: Improving Patient Care through Self-awareness and Reflection*. London, Sage.

McLeod J. (1997) *Narrative and Psychotherapy*. London, Sage.

Melia K. (1987) *Learning and Working: The Occupational Socialisation of Nurses*. London, Tavistock.

Menzies-Lyth I.E.P. (1970) *The Functioning of Social Systems as a Defence against Anxiety*. London, Tavistock.

Mills C.W. (1940) Situated actions and vocabularies of motives. *American Sociological Review* **13**, 904–909.

Mishler E.G. (1986a) *Research Interviewing: Context and Narrative*. Cambridge, Harvard University Press.

Mishler E.G. (1986b) The analysis of interview narratives. In: Sarbin T.S. (Ed.) *The Storied Nature of Human Conduct*, pp. 233–255. New York, Praeger.

Mishler E.G. (1991) *Research Interviewing: Context and Narrative*, 2nd edition. Cambridge, Harvard University Press.

Mishler E.G. (1995) Models of narrative analysis: a typology. *Journal of Narrative and Life History* **5** (2), 87–123.

Morse J. (2005) Beyond the clinical trial: expanding the criteria for evidence (Editorial). *Qualitative Health Research* **15** (1), 3–4.

Morse J. (2006) The politics of evidence. *Qualitative Health Research* **16** (3), 395–404.

Morse J.M. & Richards L. (2002) *Read Me First for a User's Guide to Qualitative Methods*. Thousand Oaks, Sage.

Mott H. & Condor S. (1997) Sexual harassment and the working lives of secretaries. In: Thomas W.I. and Kitzinger C. (Eds) *Sexual Harassment*. Buckingham, Open University Press.

Moustakas C. (1990) *Heuristic Research: Design, Methodology and Applications*. Newbury Park, Sage.

Moustakas C. (1994) *Phenomenological Research Methods*. London, Sage.

Muncey T. (2002) Individual identity or deviant case. In: Freshwater D. (Ed.) *Therapeutic Nursing*. London, Sage.

Nelson S. (2004) & McGillion M. (2004) Expertise or performance? Questioning the rhetoric of contemporary narrative use in nursing. *Journal of Advanced Nursing* **47** (6), 631–638.

Newell R. (2000) Writing academic papers: the clinical effectiveness in nursing experience. *Clinical Effectiveness in Nursing* **4**, 93–98.

Newman M. (1994) *Health as Expanding Consciousness*, 2nd edn. New York, National League for Nursing Press.

Newman M. (1999) The rhythm of relating in a paradigm of wholeness. *Image: Journal of Nursing Scholarship* **31** (3), 227–229.

NHSE (1998) *Research: What's in It for Consumers?* London, TSO.

Nielsen H.B. (1999) Black holes as sites for self-construction. In: Josselson R. & Lieblich A. (Eds) *Making Meaning of Narrative*. California, Sage.

Noy C. (2003) The write of passage: reflections on writing a dissertation in narrative methodology. *Forum Qualitative Sozialforschung/Forum: Qualitative Social Research* [On-line Journal], **4** (2). Available at: http://www.qualitative-research.net/fqs-texte/2-03/2-03noy-e.htm.

Ochberg R.L. (1996) Interpreting life stories. In: Josselson R. (Ed.) *Ethics and Process in the Narrative Study of Lives.* Thousand Oaks, Sage.

Okri B. (1997) *A Way of Being Free.* Phoenix, London.

Ollerenshaw J.A. & Creswell J.W. (2002) Narrative research: a comparison of two restorying data analysis approaches. *Qualitative Inquiry* **8** (3), 329–347.

Olson K. (2001) Using qualitative research in clinical practice. In: Morse J., Swanson J. & Kuzel A. (Eds) *The Nature of Qualitative Evidence*, pp. 259–263. Thousand Oaks, Sage.

Overcash J.A. (2004) Narrative research: a viable methodology for clinical nursing. *Nursing Forum* **39** (1), 15–22.

Parker I. (2004) Criteria for qualitative research in psychology. *Qualitative Research in Psychology* **1** (2), 95–106.

Parse R.R. (1998) *The Human Becoming School of Thought.* Thousand Oaks, Sage.

Parse R.R. (2001) The human becoming school of thought. In: Parker M. (Ed.) *Nursing Theories and Nursing Practice*. Philadelphia, F. A. Davis.

Paterson J.G. & Zderad L.T. (1976) *Humanistic Nursing.* New York, Wiley.

Patton M. (2002) *Qualitative Research and Evaluation Methods,* 3rd edn. Thousand Oaks, Sage.

Pennebaker J.W. (2000) Telling stories: the health benefits of narrative. *Literature and Medicine* **19** (1), 3–18.

PerformSocSci (2006) www.kipworld.net/.

Personal Narratives Group (1989) *Interpreting Women's Lives: Feminist Theory and Personal Narratives*. Bloomington, Indiana University Press.

Peterson C. (2004) Mothers, fathers and gender: parental narratives about children. *Narrative Inquiry* **14** (2), 323–346.

Phillips D.C. (1997) Telling the truth about stories. *Teaching and Teacher Education* **13** (1), 101–109.

Picard C. (2000) Patter of expanding consciousness in midlife women: creative movement and the narrative as modes of expression. *Nursing Science Quarterly* **13** (2), 150–157.

Polanyi N. (1962) *The Tacit Dimension.* New York, Doubleday.

Polkinghorne D.E. (1988) *Narrative Knowing and the Human Sciences.* New York, State University of New York.

Polkinghorne D.E. (1995) Narrative configuration in qualitative analysis. In: Hatch J.A. & Wisniewski R. (Eds) *Life History and Narrative*. London, Falmer Press.

Porter Abbott H. (2002) *The Cambridge Introduction to Narrative*. Cambridge, Cambridge University Press.

Predeger E. (1996) Womanspirit: a journey into healing through art in breast cancer. *Advances in Nursing Science* **18** (3), 48–58.

Priest H.M. (2000) The use of narrative in the study of caring: a critique. *NTResearch* **5** (4), 245–250.

Procter I. & Padfield M. (1999) Work orientations and women's work: a critique of Hakim's theory of the heterogeneity of women. *Gender, Work and Organization* **6**, 152–162.

Punch K.F. (2000) *Developing Effective Research Proposals*. London, Sage.

Reason P. (2003) Doing co-operative inquiry. In: Smith J. (Ed.) *Qualitative Psychology: A Practical Guide to Methods*. London, Sage.

Redman P. (2005) The narrative formation of identity revisited: narrative construction, agency and unconscious. *Narrative Inquiry* **15** (1), 25–44.

Repper J. (2000) Adjusting the focus of mental health nursing: incorporating service users' experiences of recovery. *Journal of Mental Health* **9** (6), 575–587.

Richardson L. (1990) Narrative and sociology. *Journal of Contemporary Ethnography* **19** (1), 116–135.

Ricoeur P. (1984) *Time and Narrative*, Vols 1–3. University of Chicago Press.

Riessman C.K. (1993) *Narrative Analysis*. Newbury Park, Sage.

Riessman C.K. (2006) Narrative analysis. In: Jupp V. (Ed.) *The SAGE Dictionary of Social Research Methods*, pp. 186–189. London, Sage.

Riley T. & Hawe P. (2005) Researching practice: the methodological case for narrative inquiry. *Health Education Research* **20** (2), 226–236.

Ritchie J., Lewis J. & Gillian E. (2003) Designing and selecting samples. In: Ritchie J. & Lewis J. (Eds) *Qualitative Research Practice: A Guide for Social Science Students and Researchers*, pp. 77–109. London, Sage.

Rittmann M., Rivera J. & Godwin I. (1997) Phenomenological study of nurses caring for dying patients. *Cancer Nursing* **20**, 115–119.

Roberts B. (2002) *Biographical Research*. Buckingham, Open University Press.

Rogers A.G., Casey M.E., Ekert J. et al. (1999) An interpretive poetics of languages of the unsayable. In: Josselson R. & Lieblich A. (Eds) *Making Meaning of Narratives*, pp. 77–106. Thousand Oaks, Sage.

Rogers C. (1961) *On Becoming a Person*. Boston, Houghton.

Rogers C.R. (1991) *Client-Centered Therapy*. London, Constable.

Rolfe G. (1998) *Expanding Nursing Knowledge*. Oxford, Butterworth Heinemann.

Rolfe G., Freshwater D. & Jasper M. (2001) *Critical Reflection for Nurses and the Caring Professions: A User's Guide*. Basingstoke, Palgrave.

Rose N. (1996) Psychoanalytic narratives: writing the self into contemporary cultural phenomena. *Narrative Inquiry* **13** (2), 301–315.

Rosenberg W. & Donald A. (1995) Evidence based medicine: an approach to clinical problem solving. *British Medical Journal* **310**, 1122–1126.

Rowan J. (2000) Back to basics: two kinds of therapy. *Counselling* **12** (2), 76–78.

Rowley-Jolivet E. & Carter-Thomas S. (2005) The rhetoric of conference presentation introductions: context, argument and interaction. *International Journal of Applied Linguistics* **15** (1), 45–47.

Russell G.M. & Kelly N.H. (2002) Research as interacting dialogic processes: implications for reflexivity [47 paragraphs]. *Forum Qualitative Sozialforschung/ Forum: Qualitative Social Research* [on-line journal], **3** (3). Available at: http://www.qualitative-research.net/fqs-text/3-02/3-02russellkelly-e.htm

Ryan M.L. (1993) Narrative in real time: chronicle, mimesis and plot in baseball broadcast. *Narrative* **1** (2), 138–155.

Saldaña J. (2003) Dramatizing data: a primer. *Qualitative Inquiry* **9** (2), 218–236.

Salvage J. (1998) Evidence based practice: a mixture of motives? *Nursing Times Research* **3** (6), 406–418.

Sandelowski M. (1986) The problem of rigor in qualitative research. *Advances in Nursing Science* **8** (3), 27–37.

Sandelowski M. (1991) Telling stories: narrative approaches in qualitative research. *Image, Journal of Nursing Scholarship* **23** (3), 161–168.

Sandelowski M. (1993) Rigor or rigor mortis: the problem of rigor in qualitative research revisited. *Advances in Nursing Science* **16** (2), 1–8.

Sandelowski M. (1996) Truth/story telling in nursing inquiry. In: Kikuchi J.F., Simmons H. & Romyn D. (Eds) *Truth in Nursing Inquiry*, pp. 111–124. Thousand Oaks, Sage.

Sandelowski M. & Barosso J. (2003) Writing the proposal for a qualitative methodology project. *Qualitative Health Research* **13** (6), 781–820.

Sarbin T.S. (1986) The narrative as root metaphor for psychology. In: Sarbin T.S. (Ed.) *The Storied Nature of Human Conduct*, pp. 3–21. New York, Praeger.

Savage J. (2000) One voice, different tunes: issues raised by dual analysis of a segment of qualitative data. *Journal of Advanced Nursing* **31** (6), 1493–1500.

Seale C. (1999) *The Quality of Qualitative Research*. London, Sage.

Seers K. & Milne R. (1997) Randomised controlled trials in nursing (Editorial). *Quality in Health Care* **6** (11), 1.

Sheehan J. (1986) Nursing research in Britain: the state of the art. *Nurse Education Today* **6**, 3–6.

Shenhav S.R. (2005) Thin and thick narrative analysis: on the question of defining and analyzing political narratives. *Narrative Inquiry* **15** (1), 75–99.

Silva M., Sorrell J. & Sorrell C. (1995) From Carper's patterns of knowing to ways of being: an ontological philosophical shift in nursing. *Advances in Nursing Science* **18**, 1–13.

Silverman D. (2005) *Doing Qualitative Research*, 2nd edn. London, Sage.

Smith C.P. (2000) Content analysis and narrative analysis. In: Reis H.T. & Judd C.M. (Eds) *Handbook of Research Methods in Social and Personality Psychology*, pp. 313–335. London, Cambridge University Press.

Smith D.E. (1987) *The Everyday World as Problematic. A Feminist Sociology*. Boston, Northern University Press.

Smith P. (1992) *The Emotional Labour of Nursing*. Basingstoke, Palgrave Macmillan.

Smith R. (1998) 'It doesn't count because it's subjective!'. (Re) conceptualising the role as 'validity' embraces subjectivity. Paper presented in the Advanced Paper section of the AARE Annual Conference, Adelaide.

Smythe W.E. & Murray M.J. (2000) Owning the story: ethical considerations in narrative research: *Ethics and Behaviour* **10**, 11–36.

Sparkes A. (2001) Myth 94. Qualitative health researchers will agree about validity. *Qualitative Health Research* **11** (4), 538–552.

Spence D.P. (1982) *Narrative Truth and Historical Truth: Meaning and Interpretation in Psychoanalysis*. New York, W.W. Norton and Co.

Stake R.E. (1995) *The Art of Case Study Research*. Thousand Oaks, Sage.

Stockwell F. (1972) *The Unpopular Patient*. Royal College of Nursing Research project. Series 1 no 2. London, Royal College of Nursing.

Stoddard M.C.J. (2004) Generalizability and qualitative research in the post-modern world. *Graduate Journal of Social Science* **1** (2), 303–317.

Strauss A.L. & Corbin J. (1998) *Basics of Qualitative Research: Techniques and Procedures for Developing Grounded Theory*, 2nd edn. Thousand Oaks, Sage.

Styles M. & Moccia P. (Eds) (1993) *On Nursing: A Literary Celebration*. New York, National League for Nursing Press.

Sumner M. (2006) Ethics. In: Jupp V. (Ed.) *The Sage Dictionary of Social Research Methods*. London, Sage.

Thomas W.I. & Thomas D.S. (1928) *The Child in America*. New York, Knopf.

Todres L. & Galvin K. (2005) Pursuing both breadth and depth in qualitative research: illustrated by a study of the experience of intimate caring for a loved one with Alzheimer's disease. *International Journal of Qualitative Methods* **4** (2), 1–11.

Van Maanen J. (1988) *Tales of the Field: On Writing Ethnography*. Chicago, University of Chicago Press.

Vezeau T. (1993) Use of narrative in human care enquiry. In: Gaut D. (Ed.) *A Global Agenda for Caring*. New York, National League for Nursing Press.

Vezeau T. (1994) Narrative inquiry in nursing. In: Chinn P.L. & Watson J. (Eds) *Art and Aesthetics in Nursing*. New York, National League for Nursing Press.

Walsh M. & Ford P. (1989) *Nursing Rituals, Research and Rational Actions*. Oxford, Butterworth Heinemann.

Watson M.J. & Chinn P.L. (1994) Introduction. In: Chinn P.L. & Watson M.J. (Eds) *Art and Aesthetics in Nursing*. New York, National League for Nursing Press.

Webb C. (1992) The use of the first person in academic writing: objectivity, language and gatekeeping. *Journal of Advanced Nursing* **17**, 747–752.

Webb C. (2002) Editorial: How to make your article more readable. *Journal of Advanced Nursing* **38** (1), 1–2.

Wengraf T. (2000) *Qualitative Research Interviewing: Biographic Narrative and Semi-Structured Methods*. Thousand Oaks, Sage.

Wetherell M., Taylor S. & Yates S. (2001) *Discourse Theory and Practice*. London, Sage.

White C., Woodfield K. & Ritchie J. (2003) Reporting and presenting qualitative data. In: Ritchie J. & Lewis J. (Eds) *Qualitative Research Practice: A Guide for Social Science Students and Researchers*, pp. 287–320. London, Sage.

White H. (1973) *Metahistory. The Historical Imagination in Nineteenth Century Europe*. Baltimore, Johns Hopkins University Press.

Wiltshire J. (1995) Telling a story, writing a narrative: terminology in health care. *Nursing Inquiry* **2**, 75–82.

Winter R. (2002) Truth or fiction: problems of validity and authenticity in narratives of action research. *Educational Action Research* **10** (1), 143–154.

Wolcott H. (1994) *Transforming Data: Description, Analysis and Interpretation*. Thousand Oaks, Sage.

Wolcott H. (2001) *Writing up Qualitative Research*, 2nd edn. Thousand Oaks, Sage.

Wood J. & Wilson-Barnett J. (1999) The influence of user involvement on the learning of mental health nursing students. *Journal of Research in Nursing*, **4** (4), 257–270.

Woodman M. (1985) *The Pregnant Virgin*. Toronto, Inner City Books.

Young-Mason J. (1988) *States of Exile*. New York, National League for Nursing Press.

Younger J.B. (1990) Literary works as a way of knowing. *Image* **22** (1), 39–43.

Index